"Losing a loved one to death pushes us into a series of feelings, beliefs, and behaviors that we try strongly to resist. These are painful and scary, and we fear that these experiences of our brokenness may never end. Antonio Sausys has taken [my] 'tasks of mourning' and shows how the simple practices of yoga can help us fulfill these tasks and bring us the re-integration and relief that we seek. Practicing the wisdom of this ancient mind-body discipline can help the mourner begin to integrate [his or her] experiences after loss and to re-establish a sense of wholeness."

—J. William Worden, PhD, ABPP, author of *Grief Counseling and Grief Therapy* and *Children and Grief: When a Parent Dies*

"Provides in-depth understanding of psychosomatic aspects of grief and guides us through somatopsychic methods of yoga that empower us to regain our health, inner peace, and happiness."

—**Ananda Balayogi Bhavanani**, chairman of ICYER at Ananda Ashram, Pondicherry, India, and honorary international advisor to the International Association of Yoga Therapists, USA, and various Gitananda yoga associations worldwide

"With compassion and clarity, Antonio Sausys brings dignity to the grieving process as he guides you, step-by-step, through loss to transformation and rebirth. Herein lies an important road map for the difficult rite of passage that we all must face at some point in our lives."

—**Anodea Judith**, PhD, author of *Wheels of Life: Eastern Body, Western Mind*

"In this book, Antonio shows us his skillfulness as a master teacher and skilled yoga therapist who offers us practical and accessible tools to meet the natural process of grieving. His years of experience in working with grief through his personal life and work with students shines through in this very pragmatic manual for how to heal through grief, not by leaving grief behind, but by moving all the way through it with love, kindness, and compassion for ourselves, and for what we have lost."

—**Richard Miller, PhD**, psychologist, meditation teacher of nondualism, and author of *The iRest Program for Healing PTSD* and *Yoga Nidra: The Meditative Heart of Yoga*

"A loving approach to transforming grief and loss. Antonio's work is East-West wisdom at its finest."

—**Larry Payne, PhD**, founder of Samata International Yoga and Health Institute; coauthor of *Yoga for Dummies* and *Yoga Rx and the Business of Teaching Yoga*; and director at Yoga Therapy Rx™ and Prime of Life Yoga™

"The heart of yoga is here in Antonio Sausys' *Yoga for Grief Relief*. Sausys understands grief firsthand, as well as yoga's capacity to help us heal from the inside out. Trust Sausys' deeply intuitive, compassionate, and authoritative voice as he helps you release the bodily effects of grief, guides changes in your perception, and opens you to greater self-awareness. I fully endorse this practice and this book!"

—**Amy Weintraub**, founding director of the LifeForce Yoga Healing Institute and author of *Yoga for Depression* and *Yoga Skills for Therapists*

YOGA *for* GRIEF RELIEF

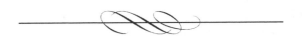

simple practices for transforming
your grieving mind & body

ANTONIO SAUSYS, MA, CMT, RYT

New Harbinger Publications, Inc.

Publisher's Note

Excerpts from *Tirukural* from WEAVER'S WISDOM by Satguru Sivaya Subramuniyaswami, copyright © 1999 Satguru Sivaya Subramuniyaswami. Reprinted by permission of Himalayan Academy.

"Physical Anatomy and the Psychic Chakras" (chart) from A CHAKRA & KUNDALINI WORKBOOK by Jonn Mumford, copyright © 1994 Jonn Mumford. Reprinted by permission of Llewellyn Publications.

Distributed in Canada by Raincoast Books

Copyright © 2014 by Antonio Sausys
        New Harbinger Publications, Inc.
        5674 Shattuck Avenue
        Oakland, CA 94609
        http://www.newharbinger.com

Cover design by Amy Shoup; Text design by Tracy Marie Carlson; Acquired by Jess O'Brien; Edited by Marisa Solis; With the creative assitance of Elliott Vogel

Library of Congress Cataloging-in-Publication Data on file

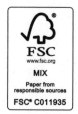 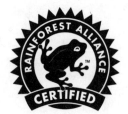

Printed in the United States of America

16   15   14

10   9   8   7   6   5   4   3   2   1   First printing

This book is dedicated to my mother, Olga Themis Marun Avisap, who, even in her passing, gave me more tools than I can comprehend to become the professional I am today. By taking me lovingly by the hand, as we pierced together through difficulties in life, she prepared me for the transformation of the grief her loss left behind into who I am today.

Her trust in me encouraged me to take on this journey; her respect for discipline gave me grounds for persevering when in doubt. I am aware she died concerned about not seeing me become the man she formed. The unstoppable force of her teachings is a testament to how, while I did lose her physical presence, she will forever be weaved into the tapestry of my heart.

Wherever you are, Mom, in whatever way you can see me, here it is....Thank you, again!

Contents

6 The Process of Transformation   129

Conclusion   151

Glossary   155

References   159

Acknowledgments

My deep gratitude goes to Lyn Prashant. Her immense knowledge of the implications of grief for the body informed and enlightened my understanding of this difficult time for the human heart. Her insightful mentorship transformed and enligthened my professional outlook. Her compassion and profound ability to hold space supported me through the transformation of my own bereavement. Her gentle yet fierce commitment to the truth of the soul moved me to levels of depth still manifesting in my life today. Her wisdom and dedication to serving others inspired my work. I'm honored to have had the opportunity to develop the seed she planted within me and I thank the universal order for having our paths meet in this lifetime.

I thank Elliott Vogel, whose patience, dedication, and creative assistance helped shape my writing while preserving my own voice. His edits translated the language of my heart into adequate words that now reach the ears of those willing to listen.

An image is worth a thousand words: My sincere thanks to Bryan Hendon, a powerful human being with a wizard in his eyes. Seeing myself through his lens gave me confidence and revealed a renewed image of myself.

Thanks to my dear wife, Katia, who supported me in so many loving and respectful ways throughout the process of writing this book. Her belief guided me back to my self-trust so that I could continue; she helped me remove the obstacles, again and again. Thank you, sweetie.

Finally, I must thank the wisdom of Yoga that, pouring through my life, turned me into a humble vehicle of the universal knowledge we all abide by.

Foreword

In 1984 I was living at the Living/Dying Project in Santa Fe, New Mexico, with my young husband, Mark. He was exploring the nature of his life and death provoked by the extreme affliction of metastasized head and neck cancer. I was newly married, and both the grieving wife and designated survivor. With Mark's death, Degriefing (Integrative Grief Therapy) was born; and my life's work was shown to me.

At first I questioned how I was going to continue to find meaning in my solo journey. I asked Mark, "Who am I? Who dies? Where do you go? What am I to do with the rest of my life?"

"Learn to love everything as you love me," was his simply stated response. I sought out professionals to help me learn to do that, and yet felt invisible, not heard, not seen. I didn't even understand how to begin to look for me. A caring and concerned friend treated me to my first experience of truly conscious body-work, which helped me begin to tolerate being in my skin.

I also noted that when I coaxed my grieving body into some yoga poses, I felt the molecular shift of my internal particles reorganizing. As an athlete, physical education teacher, and coach I saw how the physical body not only needs its own expression but actually demands physical release. This resets the balance of the many interconnected complex biological systems involved in grief. My thinking was clearer after a run, or a dance, or a swim. I saw that when I engaged my body, I felt energized rather than drained. I was feeling a life force inside of me resurging. How could this be? Was this okay? Would I lose my connection with Mark if the pain started to subside? This force, this fuel, what is it for?…To do what?… To know what? I was reappearing in a new version of my ever-changing self.

As I was preparing to graduate from the Grief Counseling Certification Program at the Graduate School of Professional Psychology at JFK University, I was offered a position as the director of the first holistic health spa in the southern cone of South America. Before departing the San Francisco Bay Area, I stated I would manifest the most amazing yoga teacher in South America. This statement actualized itself when Antonio interviewed for the position of yoga instructor on the spa staff. I shared my vision of working with the bereaved and asked if he would like to participate. His response was passionate and genuine, exhibiting continued interest, devotion, and commitment.

Yoga for Grief Relief is an offshoot of the Degriefing process, representing the work of Integrative Grief Therapy at its core. It directly relates to somatic thanatology, which uses integrative therapeutic interventions as externalizing tools involving the body, mind, and spirit. Each individual chooses and uses the tools that will help him or her navigate the unchartered waters of grief. Yoga is the master transformer by offering teaching and options for everything and everyone. Grief turns us inside out and upside down and so does yoga; compassionately, lovingly, individually, it meets us where we are in ourselves. Yoga guides us to a way of life that promotes healthy intentional change. It is a way of self-love and love for all.

I saw in Antonio the infinite possibilities and wide-ranging opportunities for him to assist the bereaved. I found that his highly skilled approach along with his expert training in both the yogic tradition and body-oriented psychotherapy provided him with a mind-body balance cosmically suited for his lifework as a yoga master. He is devoted to the highest good for everyone and is a loving and fierce taskmaster transmitting the knowledge of the yogic way of living. I knew that Antonio was the one to carry forth the Degriefing work through Yoga.

It is all here in this important book. It delicately combines and correlates the use of Eastern wisdom with Western philosophy. We are grieving globally and need a dose of universal knowledge to promote balance within each one of us.

This book is a gift, a friend, and a tool. It offers maps to demystify and normalize aspects of grieving by presenting options for transforming our physical grief, balancing systems compromised by its profound and humbling effects. Since we are jumbled, scattered, and shattered already, we are in a prime position to integrate new coping skills for a life based in the budding sense of our newly revealed personal reality.

In *Yoga for Grief Relief* we learn to express, not repress; to externalize, not internalize; to breathe again and relocate all our losses to our heart center so we can thrive within our newly met self. Antonio's work has furthered the development of Degriefing's basic premises and illuminates the process of working with our grief. Yoga provides support for all the systems and is the container for integration of mind-body-spirit.

Read and cherish this book; digest it, share it, and embody the relief you seek. With the teachings of yoga and Antonio's astute guidance, take a deep breath and buckle your psychic seat belt. You are on your way home.

—Lyn Prashant, PhD

Introduction

Grief is a radical opportunity to transform our awareness, but few of us know it. When I was twenty years old, my mother died of a stroke. For two and a half years, I lived in a state of denial, completely disconnected from my feelings. When I was finally able to be with my pain, I discovered, to my astonishment, that my body had created an additional calcium deposit between one of my ribs and the breastbone—what the body will sometimes do in response to a fracture. In essence, what my mind had been hiding, my body showed with pristine clarity: I had a broken heart.

As life continued after the loss of my mother, I began training with Lyn Prashant, an outstanding grief counselor and therapist and creator of the Degriefing process, a comprehensive mind-body approach to grief therapy. She helped me learn that grief is one of our least-tapped sources of self-knowledge. Sometime after starting to work together, Lyn asked me to develop a yoga practice to address the body-centered effects of grief, which can range from feelings of lethargy to dull aches, tightness in the chest cavity, shortness of breath, and sleeplessness. I was well equipped through my training as a somatic psychotherapist and yoga teacher. But it was my own personal experience of grief that led me to build a *sadhana*, or spiritual discipline, that eventually became a holistic practice I call Yoga for Grief Relief.

Today many of us, though we don't know it, live in a perpetual state of unacknowledged grief. There are many reasons for this. One primary reason is that we live in a society that often shies away from the powerful emotions that grief presents to us. We are often stoic, lumbering through loss without feeling; returning to work or our daily lives after the loss like nothing happened, we bury our grief deep inside of us, where it remains trapped, both in body and mind.

Grief happens in the body, yet the physical symptoms that come up in the grieving process are not always dealt with as directly as they should be. These symptoms are just as common to the grieving process as mental and emotional symptoms and require just as much attention in order to be treated. Talk therapy can be wonderful, but too often the body-centered effects of grief get subsumed under the emotional issues being dealt with. A person can, at the same time and with not much difficulty, experience relief from these physical symptoms by performing a few basic exercises. These exercises, known collectively as yoga, were developed more than six thousand years ago by people gifted in the mental powers of intuition. They realized directly what we in the West are beginning to understand today through the advent of modern science: that the human mind and body truly share a connection and influence one another, and that, through practice, one can live freely in an abundance of joy and presence of Spirit.

Abundance of joy? You may think you have picked up the wrong book, since these pages are focused on grief and the methods that can help those suffering from its effects. But I have experienced firsthand the joy yoga can provide amid the most overwhelming sorrow, the healing brought about by the performance of simple physical movements and different breathing techniques—practices you may already be familiar with. What this book offers is not a "retreat" from grief, nor a "release" from grief, but simply some *relief* from grief. Once we are able to work *physically* with the new reality loss has thrown us into, we will then be able to better understand what it is that has happened to us. Once we are able to acknowledge that, on one hand, our lives will never be the same and that, on the other hand, all the potential of the universe lies within us, a different picture starts to emerge.

Lyn Prashant affirms that "we don't get over our losses, we transform our relationship to them," and I agree with her one hundred percent. Grief is a powerful source of information about who we are, when we dare to look. There is a natural progression from one to the other, and if we are able to transform our relationship to grief in a way that results in improved self-knowledge, then we can establish a new identity. We identify ourselves through the persons and things we are attached to; when we lose them, we lose part of who we are. Yet we continue being, only in a way that is not known to us. The process of finding out who the new "one" is is multilayered. It involves understanding and dealing with the physical symptoms of grief; actually completing the grieving process; and reidentifying ourselves, not based on preconceived or prelearned notions but instead on our true essence, the one we've come so much closer to thanks to having been stripped of our previous identity. For that to happen, we must work. The *sadhana* I've developed offers a practice—the foundation for the work we must do—and along the way I'll share tools to help us reap the benefits we are after.

By sitting with awareness we start to accept the changes we are now faced with. As we consciously work with and even challenge our learned reactions, we ask: What starts to emerge from the chaos that loss leaves behind? It is a grounded individual, one who is able to accept the new reality and to continue with life, a calm practitioner, even a curious yogi. And why do we practice? It is for the same reason that people in modern-day India sat in yogic postures six thousand years ago practicing meditation: because the desire to resolve suffering is universal. We all need coping mechanisms, we all need treatments that soothe our restless minds and our aching bodies, but, above all, we need the knowledge that can be gained simply by basking in one's inner silence.

The practice I have developed for transforming grief from a painful experience into a conscious source of self-knowledge is introduced in this book in a six-part sequence: breathing exercises, body movements, cleansing techniques, relaxation, mental reprogramming, and meditation.

The breathing techniques help bring back a sense of control to the individual by manipulating the *prana*, or vital force, which helps unite the gap between the conscious and the unconscious. The body movements serve to manage the body's physical symptoms of grief, particularly addressing pain and other acute symptoms. The cleansing techniques help reset the endocrine system, affecting the fight-or-flight response, which plays an essential role in the grief reaction and the feelings associated with it. Relaxation is included with the intention of diminishing the stress levels that increase during grief. The powerful yogic principle of Resolve helps reset mental patterns and focuses the mind toward the transformation of grief. Finally, meditation is used to address the Spirit: once the body is still and the mind is calm, that which is neither body nor mind can manifest more clearly.

The main *asana* (physical posture) of the Yoga for Grief Relief practice is called the Windmill. Symbolically, the windmill serves as an analogy for the process of transformation of grief into a new identity. The forces of the unknown—the wind—power the mechanisms of the windmill, just as the mystery of loss creates a churning in the depths of our own selves. As the windmill utilizes the sometimes wild and destructive force of wind energy to mechanically transform hard grains into edible flour, the techniques in this *sadhana* can transform our Spirits, left vacant by loss but open to receiving the knowledge that exists within us. Just as the grain being pulverized results in a finer quality of flour, the yoga exercises shared here operate at a neurochemical level, improving our mood and strengthening our resolve in the face of insurmountable loss. Not only does the physical component of the practice make us feel better, new patterns are established that link the conscious performance of certain exercises with an overall sense of well-being. More neuroscientists are discovering that our brains are resilient organs, capable of far more than we had previously given them credit for, especially in the realm of emotional disorders and addiction. But the conclusions of modern neuroscience all seem to point to one essential truth of biological determinism: practice makes perfect. Our brains are capable of reformation, but they require discipline. Yoga is an ancient art, one whose founders realized the importance of practice for physical results in the body, lasting impressions of tranquility in the mind, and the evolution of the soul.

It is the techniques themselves that are the inspiration for this book. The practice—and its effects—resonates strongly in my life today and in those of my students who have engaged in it. The aim of this practice is to help you accept the reality of loss and then work through the pain of grief. Once a person can adjust to this new situation or environment without the loved one, then he or she can emotionally reinvest the love attached to the lost person or object and embark on a new life.

When later on in life my father passed away, despite my knowledge of the grieving process and the awareness I have about what practices can help traverse it, nothing could save me from experiencing—again—that deep pain of loss. There is no way around grief; going through it is the only healthy way. This book and the techniques I demonstrate here are not a way of "getting over grief." Instead of avoiding the feelings, these techniques are designed to help you navigate through emotions that are not always pleasant. Because of my experience as a yoga therapist, I had an awareness of what some of my reactions were going to be when my father died, and I knew I had tools I could utilize to help normalize those reactions and emerge anew. It is my hope that this book will offer a window to the unique way you experience your own grief, and give you some simple techniques that will help you safely explore that experience.

You may benefit from reading this book if you are looking to explore or work with grief in the intimacy of a home yoga practice or existing studio workout, if you would like to complement the grief therapy that you are already engaged in, or if you work with grieving individuals in your profession and would like to integrate the knowledge of yoga into your existing toolbox.

In chapter 1, you will find information that will help normalize your grief. You will start to understand the uniqueness of your grieving process and, at the same time, acknowledge some universal truths about it. In chapter 2, you will learn some of the succinct wisdom of yoga, which will help you understand grief in a different cultural context and how particular energy centers (chakras) react when we grieve. The wisdom teachings are a knowledge that is in action in all of us, regardless of our backgrounds or belief systems.

In chapter 3, you will learn about each general category of practice and how they can be used to address different aspects of the grieving process. Chapter 4 presents the exercises in a simple how-to manner, including how each technique can help transform grief. Chapter 5 offers guidance on how to set up your practice according to what's possible for you and what your personal intention is. This chapter also shows you how to start framing your ideal conditions for practice, identifying what you want to accomplish along with any possible barriers. In any case, what's most important is that you meet yourself where you are. It may sound simple but is often a challenge for those faced with loss.

After learning the techniques and starting to plan how to integrate them into your life, you will discover how the yoga practice serves the greater process of transformation that awakens your spiritual connection with life. In chapter 6, you will learn to identify old patterns and ways of thinking you would like to discard, and promote those you now welcome as part of the journey toward your most complete version of yourself. Though you might not yet have finished grieving, you can start to see ways in which the experience of grief serves to transform your life by getting to the core of who you really are.

As you read through this book, remember to be gentle with yourself. Use this book as a guide; draw from it when needed, and remember that in order to be effective, these techniques need to be practiced. Intellectual information is not what we are after. If our minds could solve the mystery of loss and grief, you would not be reading this book, nor would I have written it. I hope that in reading this book, and through your own practice, you may access the hidden gift that lies trapped in the painful experience of grief.

CHAPTER 1

Grief: A Normal Response to Loss

Grief affects the physical, mental, spiritual, and emotional aspects of our humanity. It is our normal reaction to loss, but this truism does not make it any easier to deal with. We seem to live as if the things we are attached to are always going to be there. And many of us were raised in cultures that do not openly acknowledge grief. When faced with the pain and shock of loss we feel awkward, clueless and confused, overwhelmed, and unprepared to begin to soothe ourselves. A phrase heard frequently from grieving people is, "I feel as if I am going crazy." Some consider the process of bereavement to be an illness, rather than a normal part of the human condition that seeks outlet and expression. The cries of heartbreak allow the body to achieve balance by facilitating the release of stress hormones and soothing some of the physical pain encountered in grief.

People experience grief in different ways. We experience a vast array of emotional and physical symptoms, from the agitated and anxious to the lethargic and depressed, from body aches and muscle stiffness to disruptions in sleeping and eating habits. The common factor in all these symptoms is how our brains are involved in the grieving process. Current research exploring the role that the brain plays in emotional life is discussed later in this chapter in "Grief and the Brain."

Yoga for Grief Relief is an entire program designed to support and inform you in all aspects of bereavement. It's important to recognize that while the grieving process is profoundly uncomfortable, it is actually normal. However, *complicated grief* that continues to provoke unhealthy behaviors over the long term and that takes an extreme toll on the griever is often better served by professional help.

Defining Grief: The Western View

Grief is a pervasive force endemic to the human condition, and an essential part of our emotional makeup. Each culture relates to grief uniquely. Where you grew up, how open was your society to discussing issues that produce grief? What common funerary rituals did your culture provide? What values were extolled by your family? Did people in your life typically die at home or in hospitals? Did you grow up in a large household or are you an only child?

The answers to these questions can and often do significantly influence reactions to loss. Just think of how a griever may experience his or her sorrow differently if in Uruguay or in the United States. It is the custom in Uruguay that family and close friends spend the night with the mourner immediately after a death to share the pain and sorrow, staying awake thanks to a few cups of coffee. Then, together, they say farewell to the deceased and put the remains to rest. In the United States, a more common way of accompanying a mourner is to attend a wake, an event that occurs sometime after the death, in which people tell funny stories, mention good qualities of the one gone, and then celebrate the deceased's life lavishly with alcohol and food.

Also consider an individual living in a society that sets aside a special day for remembering and celebrating the dead, versus a person living in a culture that finds the outward exposure of sorrow socially inappropriate and lacking taste. These cultural differences also affect the opinions, views, and beliefs of Western psychologists and clinicians, who often assume very contradictory views to those of the monks and swamis I trained with during my initiation to yoga.

My dual training in the fields of somatic psychotherapy and the timeless wisdom of Yoga has allowed me to experience both worldviews firsthand.

Regrettably, Western culture tends to sweep grief under the rug by ignoring it entirely or compartmentalizing it. Only minimal attention to grief is allowed, effectively preventing us from understanding its nature. It is skillful to ask ourselves questions such as, "What is the first great loss I remember suffering? Who could I talk to? How did I cope with the experience? How did the people around me act?" This inquiry encourages self-awareness and understanding of how your family and cultural background influence your relationship to your own grief today.

Despite the rich variety of answers to these questions, I would like to start by saying that grief is our *natural* response to loss—any loss. Traditionally, we think of grief as being the range of emotional and psychological responses experienced after the death of someone we love. But death is not the only type of loss that elicits grief. Some might feel grief over the loss of a prized possession, a pet, a job, a dream, or their youth. In fact, I have witnessed humans grieving the loss of perceived invincibility after breaking a bone, the discontinuation of a regularly scheduled TV show or a favorite brand of sneakers, or having reached the end of a delicious novel. The combined effects of our losses, big and small, major and minor, accumulate in our bodies. The judgment that some losses are trivial, and are therefore unimportant to consider, can exacerbate feelings of confusion, isolation, and shame. This can interfere with a griever's ability to accept the reality of where he or she is in his or her personal process.

Two Types of Losses

Identifying primary and secondary losses is helpful for compassionate self-reflection. The initial loss, the one that occurs first, is usually referred to as the *primary loss*. Losses that occur as a result of this underlying primary loss are known as *secondary losses*.

Primary losses are more easily identified, while the secondary ones can be more subtle and perhaps underacknowledged with regard to their profound emotional intensity. For example, a woman whose marriage ends in divorce (primary loss) who then suffers the exclusion of events previously found on her social calendar (secondary loss) is dealing with the exponential effects of the combined losses. Perhaps her ex-husband is still being invited to events, or perhaps her coupled friends are uncomfortable with her new single status. The secondary loss named here is the loss of her social network.

It is important to acknowledge that while each primary loss occurs only once, secondary losses may continue to occur and are therefore experienced frequently. In the previous example, the woman experienced the divorce only once, but the loss of her social network is felt every time she is not invited out by "their" friends. In addition, the burden of assuming roles and responsibilities formerly handled by her ex—such as paying the mortgage bill, checking the air in the tires, or managing the household in ways she has not had to before—is a constant, painful reminder of all that has been lost since the divorce. The secondary loss continually retriggers her grief due to the primary loss of the husband.

In another example, losing all of one's family heirlooms in a house fire (primary loss) might evoke the experience of severing one's ancestral past (secondary loss). Secondary losses aren't always recognized as valid causes of grief, but they can bring on tremendous sorrow and repeatedly reignite the pain that was experienced from the primary loss.

Symptoms of Grief

Although no two individuals grieve in the same way, there is some consistency in the emotional, physical, and mental symptoms associated with the grieving process. Some of the most commonly acknowledged feelings that relate to grief can be seen in the following table (adapted with permission from Lunche, 1999):

EMOTIONAL SYMPTOMS OF GRIEF

- Shock, numbness

- Sadness

- Emptiness

- Feeling helpless

- Feeling out of control

- Anger

- Guilt, regret

- Resentment

- Depression

- Loneliness, longing, yearning

- Fear, anxiety, insecurity

- Feelings of betrayal, disloyalty

- Diminished self-concern

- Sorrow for the one who died

- Desire to join the deceased

- Suicidal feelings

Table 1: Emotional symptoms of grief

Even though sadness is the feeling most commonly expressed while grieving, a wide range of emotions is often determined by the quality of the relationship we had with what's been lost, as well as by the circumstances surrounding the loss. As you can see from the Emotional Symptoms of Grief table, the impact of our grief may present many complex combinations of emotions affecting us distinctly.

One example of this might be when an abusive husband dies—the wife could feel more relieved than sad. When a father commits suicide, the children he left behind may be coping with their shame and anger more than with depression. In my personal and professional experience, when a relationship that was more positive ends, feelings of depression are very likely to surface. Whereas the more conflicted a relationship is, the greater the likelihood is that anger and guilt will appear.

My father and I finally developed a pristine friendship after many years of not getting along. What soothed my heart most after he passed were the nurturing memories of our newly established friendship. Because we painstakingly attended to all our unfinished business, I could grieve his loss without regret or ambivalence. Being at that point in our relationship at the time of his passing permitted me to connect with the more profoundly painful and challenging aspects of my grief process and be present to experience the emotionally joyous and pleasant memories bubbling up inside me.

Four Tasks of Mourning: A Road Map for the Grieving Process

Grief presents us with tremendous duality. We grieve both uniquely, according to our life's variables, and universally, as all humans do. Leaders in the field have noted specific elements of grieving, suggesting they need to be addressed in order to fulfill a normal process. Some of them name these elements as "stages," others as "phases," of grief. Both terms suggest to me something more stale or passive in nature. Of all thinkers, J. William Worden (2009) offers the model I find best suited to the yogic ideal of practice. In his model, he names these elements "tasks," a term that clearly denotes the dynamism the process really involves. It provides an active way to move through grief's common emotional states. Worden's Four Tasks of Mourning are:

- **To accept the reality of the loss.** Accepting the reality of the loss, to Worden, implies recognizing that "reunion with the departed is impossible, at least in this life" (39). Worden describes a searching behavior that is common at this level of grieving, whereby a grieving person might "see" the deceased walking in a crowd and recognize her, only then to be confronted with the reminder of her death. Various degrees of denial could be involved in order to avoid accepting the reality of the loss.

- **To process the pain of grief.** The second task involves consciously working with the pain of grief. Worden states, "It is necessary to acknowledge and work through this pain or it can manifest itself through physical symptoms or some form of aberrant behavior" (44). This second task of mourning is of special significance to yoga because of the connection with conscious work and dedicated practice.

- **To adjust to a world without the deceased.** Worden identifies three areas of adjustment that are to be reckoned with after the loss of a loved one. *External adjustments* relate to how coping with loss affects our everyday life (e.g., what do we do with the working hours when we've just lost a job?). *Internal adjustments* refer to how death affects self-definition, self-esteem, and one's sense of self-efficacy (e.g., how can a spouse feel like a whole self again after losing his partner?). *Spiritual adjustments* imply dealing with the challenges of our belief systems and values as death shakes the foundation of one's assumptions of the world (e.g., the faithful believer questioning the existence of a just God after feeling that his prayers have not been heard).

- **To find an enduring connection with the deceased in the midst of embarking on a new life.** Worden asserts that it is essential that the mourner find new ways to continue honoring the deceased, while still remaining focused on creating a new life. Freud (1953) describes the mental process of mourning as summoning mental images of the lost loved one, detaching the previously invested love, and reestablishing the freedom of the mind. Worden suggests that we do not entirely recycle the emotional energy previously invested: he cites current research that states that maintaining an active awareness of the deceased person provides comfort and strength to the bereaved.

Although each task is essential to the process of mourning, the tasks themselves are not linear. After completing all four we may be prompted to revisit any or each of them.

Most of our efforts dealing with grief are geared toward avoiding suffering from the unusually immense pain loss inflicts on us. It is Dr. Worden's opinion that the fulfillment of all Four Tasks of Mourning is essential to promote a healthy and normal grieving process. Otherwise, we may fall into what is considered a *complicated grieving process.* In some cases, an individual's grief reaction is prolonged, becoming an almost chronic condition that may never be fully resolved.

Examining examples of complicated grief, we often see the actual manifestation of symptoms showing up at a much later time in response to a more recent, unexpected loss. This exaggerated reaction can manifest as, or turn into, a specific mental condition, such as clinical depression. In others, the grief appears disguised by symptoms and behaviors that, while seemingly unrelated to grief, are actually examples of "masked" grief (Worden 2009). It is important to differentiate these markers of complicated grief from the natural way in which grief occurs down the line: coming back unexpectedly, at times in relation to life events and other times seemingly random, and presenting us with feelings and symptoms of the old grief. This concept is well expressed in the work of Therese Rando, who coined the term STUG: Sudden Temporary Upsurge of Grief (1993).

Grief triggers grief. Fresh loss naturally triggers memories, feelings, and symptoms related to a previous loss. Sometimes we are truly shocked at the tremendous intensity of our feelings. When others who are close to us experience loss, it can easily trigger our own grief and cause us to revisit old losses even if we feel we have dealt with them already. Perhaps this is a reason why people recoil from hearing about another's grief or become uncomfortable when they witness people exhibit their grief openly. Counselors, therapists, and hospice workers who work with grief regularly see their own grief retriggered and can suffer from the effects of "caregiver's burden."

Regardless of how our grief originates, the key element is that in order to grieve a loss we need to have developed a strong emotional connection with what has been lost or what it represents to us. We need to have formed an attachment.

Attachment: The True Root of Grief

"Attachment" is generally defined as a feeling that binds someone to a person, thing, cause, or ideal. This is a remarkably similar description to what Freud stated when describing the object of grief during mourning (Freud 1953). Psychology views attachment as "an evolved behavioral system designed to regulate infants' proximity to a protector and thereby maximize chances for survival," according to John Bowlby (Diamond 2001, 277). Later on, studies conducted by Mary Ainsworth concluded that there are three major styles of attachment: secure, ambivalent-insecure, and avoidant-insecure (Broberg 2000).

Researchers Main and Solomon (1986) added a fourth style known as disorganized-insecure attachment. These early attachment styles can help predict behaviors later in life, especially adult romantic love. For example, when an individual is able to gain comfort from his parents as a child ("secure attachment"), he tends to have good self-esteem as an adult. On the other hand, when a child does not gain much comfort or contact from his parents ("avoidant attachment"), he develops adult behaviors that invest little or no emotion in social and romantic relationships.

In short, our early attachments constitute our first awareness of those who love and care for us, and influence how we love as adults. No matter what attachment style we develop, we are all like these infants—seeking survival, clinging to what is familiar. Like a packet of food coloring released into a pitcher of water, we can see our attachments permeate the substance of our life. Attachment is at the core of how we form families and how our larger social network functions. For us in the West, attachment is tantamount to love: "If I love you, I am attached to you being here forever." This association is so strong that actions indicating detachment are usually seen as a sign of a lack of love.

Our attachments inform us when we feel at home, when we are lonely, and when we are in danger. Even at a chemical level, the bonds we make with human beings and other objects affect us. When these bonds break, we can investigate the psychophysiological effects and normalize the many somatic aspects of grief manifesting as physical symptoms. Now let's discover what the perspective of psychophysiology can bring to our understanding of grief.

Grief and the Brain

How does the body express what the heart and mind are going through? Currently, there is not enough measurable scientific data on grief, and further research is still needed. Most of the existing information focuses on victims of trauma. Although all trauma involves grief, it is important to remember that not all grief is traumatic. Western psychology usually views the body as an afterthought, proclaiming that the grieving process happens mainly in our minds. More recent research in the areas of psychology, immunology, and endocrinology reveals data that shows how emotional processes like grief affect more than just our mental functioning. Psychophysiology shows how life-changing events influence virtually every area of a person's physical and mental constitution, from thought patterns to emotional well-being, immune function, and overall health (Rosenbaum and Varvin 2007; Ulvestad 2012; Van den Berg et al. 2012). Western science is just now discovering and documenting connections formulated ages ago from the meditative observations of practicing yogis. The evidence of the mind-body connections discovered by these scientists is truly fascinating, and its impact in the area of grief work is only beginning to be felt.

Two of the main symptoms associated with grieving are pain in the chest muscles and disruptions of the circadian rhythms, particularly the sleep cycle. People experience a variety of symptoms that usually change as the grieving process unfolds. What should be eminently clear from the following table (adapted with permission from Lunche, 1999) is that grief affects the body.

PHYSICAL SYMPTOMS OF GRIEF

- Pain

- Feeling of tightness in the chest

- Feeling of tightness in the throat

- Alterations in the breathing patterns (shortness of breath, frequent sighing)

- Fatigue, exhaustion, low energy

- Sleep pattern disruption (insomnia or excessive sleep)

- Eating pattern disruption (overeating or anorexia)

- Alteration of the cardiac rhythms (bradycardia, tachycardia, arrhythmia)

- Digestive system upset

- Generalized tension

- Restlessness, irritability

- Increased sensitivity to stimuli

- Dry mouth

Table 2: Physical symptoms of grief

Grief is mainly orchestrated by the limbic system. It's a central structure within the nervous system deeply involved in the way we experience emotions. The limbic system initially gathers sensory information about an experience and compares that information with previously stored knowledge, housing memories of past similar experiences, our belief systems, and cultural values. It then assigns the experience an emotional tone and integrates a response. Then the outermost sheet of neuronal tissue in the brain, the neocortex, processes the experience further and assigns meaning to it on a deeper level.

Alterations of the normal functions of the limbic system result in

- irritability,

- moodiness,

- depression,

- negative thinking,

- negative perspective,

- sleep and appetite disorders,

- social isolation,

- decreased or increased sexual drive, and

- motivation.

Many of the items on this list of mood disturbances and other symptoms are classic features of a normal grieving process, solidifying the case for the limbic system's involvement. When taking a look at other mental and social symptoms of grief, this connection with the functions of the limbic system becomes even clearer:

Mental Symptoms of Grief	Social Symptoms of Grief
• Negative anticipatory thinking	• Being isolated by others
• Disbelief	• Withdrawing from social activities
• Confusion	• Diminished desire for social activities
• Disorientation	• Coping with labels like "widowed," "single," etc.
• Absentmindedness	• Hiding grief by taking care of others
• Forgetfulness	• Losing friends, making new friends
• Poor concentration	
• Distraction	
• Difficulty focusing and attending	
• Low motivation	
• Expecting to see the deceased	
• Expecting the deceased to call	
• Preoccupation with the deceased	
• Feeling the need to tell and retell the story surrounding the loss	
• Dreams or images of the deceased	
• Denial	
• Thinking about other deaths and losses	

Table 3: Mental and social symptoms of grief (adapted with permission from Lunche, 1999)

According to Dr. James Gardner, "Grief begins in the brain" and affects the brain "from the highest cortical centers and temporal lobes to the deeper, more primitive structures in the limbic system." For our neurotransmitters, the building blocks of the brain that are essential for intercellular communication, grief "affects the way we process some of these chemicals," including the neuropeptides (2002, 6).

On a biochemical level, we react as though our entire existence is being threatened. According to Gardner, "As the serotonin system is weakened by the emotional stress of loss, the anxiety response is triggered" (2002, 6). He goes on to say that the body's fight-or-flight reaction includes the release of adrenaline. The release of hormones increases heart rate and blood pressure; stressful signals activate the endocrine glands and affect the heart, stomach, various muscle groups, and the blood vessels themselves. Other symptoms include the cooling of the extremities, pupil dilation, tremors, sweating, and nausea due to hyperventilation. Taking its cues from the brain, the body reacts to the full force of the loss as a menacing danger, a direct threat to our survival.

Neuroplasticity and Its Implications for Grief

Even though grief is seemingly an omnipresent challenge influencing our brain chemistry, we might consider the following news to be positive. Neuroplasticity refers to the brain's ability to change its structure and function in response to experience, training, and practice. In the twentieth century, our brains were thought to develop within a critical period during early childhood, and to then remain relatively immutable. This thinking meant that once we passed the critical period of development we were basically stuck in those ways, forever hardwired, fixed in form and function. This belief lowered expectations about the value of rehabilitation for those who had suffered brain injury from a stroke, for example.

Because psychiatric conditions are related to specific neuronal pathways in the brain, this also meant that once developed, a mental illness would be almost impossible to treat successfully (Begley 2007). Sharon Begley, a journalist who reports on current trends on health and science, wrote in *Time* magazine, "There was good reason for lavishly illustrated brain books to show the function, size and location of the brain's structures in permanent ink." This prevailing view also reinforced limited mental perceptions. It was simply a brain-determined reality that, after losing one's house, one might never feel truly at home again; or after losing a spouse, one could never find love again.

These beliefs have been challenged by findings that reveal that many functions of the brain remain plastic even into adulthood. Substantial changes have been documented showing that an individual can consciously and profoundly alter the way his or her neurons are activated in response to experience. These alterations affect both the brain's physical anatomy and functional organization, signifying that the brain can and does change.

"Neurons That Fire Together, Wire Together"

This is a common saying in the field of neuroscience. New connections between nervous cells are formed as we engage in different activities. These new neuronal pathways are strengthened when we repeat those activities, wiring the nervous cells together. The more we repeat these activities, the more permanent the connections become.

Even though these findings relate to how the brain compensates for injury and disease, this mechanism applies to brain activity in general. Neuroplasticity makes personal growth and development possible by allowing the nerve cells in the brain to adjust their activities in response to new situations and changes in their environment. Although this process is automatic and happens independently, outside the realm of conscious intention, we can in fact enhance the sought-after results by increasing conscious practice. The more practice, the more ingrained or imprinted the new connections become.

Research conducted on musicians by neuroscientist Alvaro Pascual-Leone, a professor of neurology at Harvard University, indicates that while the process is triggered by actual practice, mere thought can also alter the physical structure and function of our gray matter (2001). He found that the increased brain surface activated in subjects after practicing an instrument was equal to those who "thought" of the scales to be practiced. This revelation is important when understanding grief because it validates the use of techniques such as *Sankalpa*, or Resolve, which uses repetition of statements that reflect a desired state of being to induce the brain to remap itself toward such a reality.

The Brain's Insatiable Quest for Happiness

A special area of interest for those performing current research in neuroscience has been studying the brains of Buddhist monks during meditation to observe whether there is any measurable change in brain activity with the use of contemplative practices. In order to understand how our brains conduct our insatiable quest for happiness, something the monks are believed to experience thanks to meditation, Richard Davidson, a neuroscientist at the University of Wisconsin at Madison, conducted studies to find out if we can think of emotions, moods, and states such as compassion as mental skills that could somehow be ingrained in a person through training. When comparing the activity in the brains of the group of monks versus those of a control group who did not meditate, the most striking difference was in an area in the left prefrontal cortex, believed to be the site of activity that signals happiness (Davidson 2012). While the monks were generating feelings of compassion, activity in the left prefrontal cortex swamped activity in the right prefrontal cortex to a degree never before seen from purely mental activity. (The right prefrontal cortex is associated with negative moods.) On the other hand, the individuals belonging to the control group showed no such differences between the left prefrontal cortex and the right. According to Davidson, this suggests that the positive state is a skill that can be learned.

Practice Reshapes Your Brain

The new understanding of neuroplasticity related to the power of the mind's ability to change our brains promises something fundamental for the understanding of grief. By employing intentional and conscious physical and mental practice, we can change our relationship to ourselves during our emotionally fluctuating grieving process. Each action we perform, each thought we think, each word we speak then becomes an arrow shot into the field of manifestation, an opportunity for a new connection in the brain to modify the old and emphasize the establishment of a new identity.

While the focus of this book is not brain biology or neurochemistry, it is important to understand just how strong a force grief is. Regarding our mental and emotional landscape, we now comprehend that our emotional life is informed by the thoughts we think; by how the brain itself reacts to experiences, instructing our bodies to behave. You now see how many of the symptoms of grief directly relate to how our brains react when facing loss. Recall how the attachments to people from the earliest stages of our life formulate our psychic basis for the adult emotions of love and compassion. Loss is a real material experience, affecting us at every layer of our existence. The following table (adapted with permission from Lunche, 1999) indicates profound changes in behaviors when we are grieving. As we deepen our understanding of how our brains serve as the basis for many of these symptoms, we can normalize profound changes that are powerfully altering reality as we knew it.

BEHAVIORAL SYMPTOMS OF GRIEF

- Crying (sometimes unexpectedly)

- Searching for the deceased

- Carrying special objects

- Going to the grave site

- Making and keeping an altar

- Keeping belongings intact

- Looking at photos or videos of the deceased

- Listening to audio recordings of the deceased

- Talking to the deceased

- Avoiding situations that arouse grief

- Changes in daily routine

- "Staying busy"

- Assuming mannerisms of the deceased

Table 4: Behavioral symptoms of grief

By getting a sense of how intensely all systems are involved in the bereavement process, it becomes more evident that engaging certain yoga exercises intended to unite mind and body are effective in bringing back a sense of cohesion and personal control in times of grief. Through breath work, physical movements, and specific techniques designed to, for example, help reset the functioning of the endocrine system, we can take this information about grief and put it to good use. We can apply tools to integrate conscious responses that help our brains reshape themselves in an active and insightful way. Yoga helps us to be more present for our feelings of grief and it is, perhaps, the most complete body of practical knowledge you can seek out.

We will now look at what this ancient discipline expresses as to why we grieve and how grief relates to its precursor, attachment.

CHAPTER 2

Yoga and Grief

Yoga's quest to resolve human suffering is probably as old as the discipline itself. Since yoga's entrance into mainstream Western culture, it has been tailored to meet the needs of a variety of practitioners. Western styles and modulations of yoga have complemented the ancient original schools, or branches. One of the results of this diversification has been the emergence of *yoga therapy*. This system is perfectly designed for the application of yoga's teachings, philosophy, and unique methods for addressing and transforming personal imbalances manifesting as diseases or disorders. Even though other disciplines such as *yoga chikitsa* and Ayurveda deal with the therapeutic process, yoga therapy is actually more helpful in addressing the grieving process in the body, mind, and spirit.

I have come to understand grief as one of the most prevailing and unacknowledged feelings in the human heart through my personal and professional experiences. As a yogi I recognize the need for a more Spirit-centered approach to dealing with grief. Witnessing the effects on my students, along with my personal experience of practicing yoga for many years, has given me a deep understanding of yoga's effectiveness in treating grief.

Initially, yoga helps us to manage some of the physical and emotional symptoms of grief. As one's practice deepens, yoga offers profound insights into the difference between the suffering intrinsic to grief and that of attachment, which

I call the precondition for grief. Let's examine some philosophical underpinnings of yoga and how they can demystify our relationship to grief.

The Five Spokes on the Wheel of Suffering

The first extant written work on yoga that presents a comprehensive philosophy on the nature of suffering and how to alleviate it is *The Yoga Sutras of Patanjali* (Bryant 2009). In this text, attachment—the precondition for grief—is named as one of the five root causes of suffering that inevitably lead to pain and confusion. Together they are

- ignorance of the truth,

- egoism,

- attachment,

- aversion, and

- fear of death.

Ignorance of the truth refers to ignoring the essential rules that the universe abides by. An example of this is to expect a flower to be born fully bloomed, then develop backward, decreasing in size until it becomes a seed. This misapprehension can be seen as a metaphor of life in general: all living organisms have a definite beginning and a period of development, and then meet their end. Therefore, anyone contesting the flower's organic nature promotes personal suffering.

Egoism refers to false identification with the mind and body exclusively and ignoring the Spirit. The nature of both body and mind is one of craving. The body craves heat, food, touch, and rest; the mind craves acknowledgment, identification, and seeks change. Once any of our needs become satisfied, then immediately the next one kicks in. The Spirit, conversely, needs nothing because it contains everything and is the source of everything. By including our Spirit in our identification, we gain contact with an aspect of ourselves that is satisfied, truly and completely (Satyananda 1976).

Attachment refers to our dependency on the permanence of a person's presence or an object's continued availability to produce and sustain our happiness. Attachment comes from the positive experiences we have in life and the memories we form in association with them. Since all things are by their true nature absolutely impermanent, our suffering is ensured when things disappear or die. Of the five causes of suffering, attachment has a particularly important role in grief and is therefore discussed further in the following section.

Aversion is the opposite of attachment and is derived from negative experiences in life. It refers to things we don't like, prompting us to turn away from them. Because the likelihood of all things happening is evenly spread across the spectrum of reality, things we don't like will inevitably occur—and we suffer yet again.

Fear of death refers to a feeling human beings experience as part of their emotional makeup. Because death is inevitable, fearing it is a sure ticket to suffering. Regardless of how or when, we instinctively know what we fear will arrive at some point.

These five causes of suffering become like a wheel in a hamster cage. Like naive hamsters, we hurl the wheel into perpetual motion, running toward no end. If we choose to ignore the essential truth, we become identified with our bodies and minds only. This leads us to generate attachments and aversions, the ultimate being aversion to our own death, ignoring the truth that we too will inevitably die.

In *Four Chapters on Freedom*, Swami Satyananda's commentary on *The Yoga Sutras of Patanjali*, we are told that our "desire for life" is "sustained by its own force" (1976, 154). It is because of an attachment to our physical body, the swami says, that we cling to life and fear natural processes like disease and death. Since grief appears as a result of losing those things or persons we are attached to, *The Yoga Sutras* can explain the intimate relationship between grief and suffering. I am not suggesting that if we could somehow eliminate attachment our lives would be problem-free and all suffering would end. The four other causes are equally potent and important. Could simply envisioning the elimination of suffering bring some ease to our minds? By just being conscious of the five causes of suffering, we combat the initial barrier of ignorance that prevents us from knowing our true selves.

Attachment: Its Special Role for Grievers

The negative implications of attachment are quite difficult for us humans to comprehend. Why is dealing with attachment so difficult? We form attachments to perpetuate the comfort and safety we are accustomed to receive from the things and persons we attach to. Yet, we can never know just how long those things or persons will remain. Forming attachments seems to be inherent in the human condition.

Yoga addresses this uncertainty and invokes the universal truth that "All things come to an end." This calms the mind's craving for knowledge and provides an answer to the yearning question many grievers ask themselves after a loss: Why?

When we form attachments, we are relying on the permanence of things. When those things vanish, the result for us is a predictable one: we suffer. In the epic Indian tale of the Bhagavad Gita, prince Arjuna turns to his charioteer Krishna for counsel on the battlefield. While seemingly just advising the warrior on military strategy, Lord Krishna actually imparts deep spiritual wisdom to the unknowing seeker. He identifies attachment as the beginning of a chain reaction of turbulent emotions:

> "While contemplating the objects of the senses, a person develops attachment for them, and from such attachment lust develops, and from anger lust arises."
>
> —Verse 62 (1972, 122)

> "From anger, complete delusion arises, and from delusion bewilderment of memory. When memory is bewildered, intelligence is lost, and when intelligence is lost one falls down again into the material pool."
>
> —Verse 63 (1972, 123)

This explanation of how attachment manifests in human beings is an illumination from a realized master, such as Krishna, to the aspiring yogi (Bhaktivedanta 1972). This sage wisdom applies to every one of us who is learning and aspiring here on Earth. For mothers whose heightened attachment with their infants is directly connected to the continued survival of their offspring, envisioning a life of nonattachment seems nearly impossible. For most of humanity that is also true. Yet, yoga offers us pure knowledge that applies to life within the framework of what is feasible for each one of us. Yoga does not just rely on philosophy, however, to explain why we grieve; it pinpoints grief in *anahata* chakra, a specific place in the body.

Exploring the Chakras and How They Relate to Grief

The Sanskrit word *chakra* translates to "wheel" in English. This evokes an image of swirling energy, the stirring of emotional and psychic contents. The seven chakras configure a pathway moving from primal emotions and sensations (fear, anger, disgust) to love and compassion and spiritual connection.

According to yoga philosophy, human beings are in a state of continuous evolution. This evolution is symbolized by the spiraling movement of *kundalini*, an invisible energy that, when awakened, flows upward from the base of the spine to the top of the head (Satyananda 1985). During its course, this energy makes contact with several psychic centers (chakras), each of which signifies different stages in our journey toward complete selfhood. John Selby states that each chakra corresponds to a major endocrine gland, a main autonomic nerve or group of nerves and the functions they regulate within the body, and a specific manifestation or aspect of human consciousness (1992).

The chakra system is a brilliant map for understanding the connection between mind, body, and spirit. It offers a diagnostic tool as well as a field of operation for understanding and managing some of the difficult emotions involved in grief. Getting in touch with these emotions unveils aspects of the potential life lessons hidden in the symptoms we are experiencing. We begin making connections between the sensations we feel in our bodies and how our thinking is affected by such sensations. Witnessing how the three essential parts of ourselves—the mental, the physical, and the spiritual—interact, we are able to see that each thought and emotion has a correlate within our physical body. This recognition facilitates our journey of integration and evolution of consciousness.

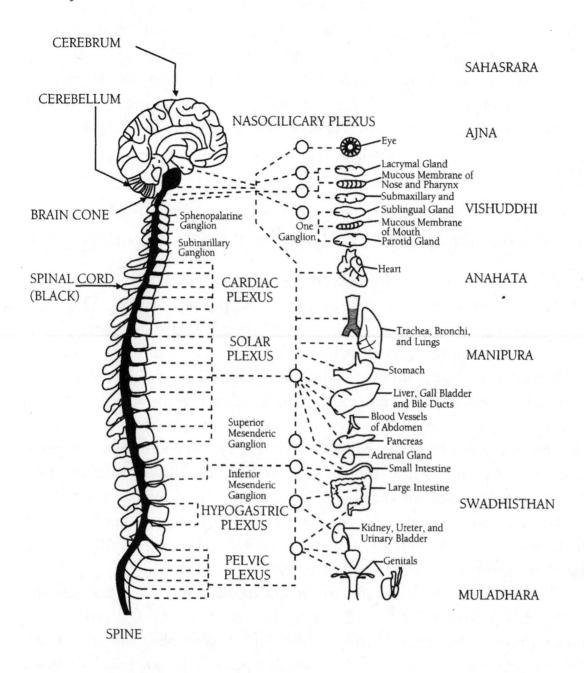

ROOT CHAKRA: THE SURVIVOR

The first chakra (*mooladhara*) is located at the pelvic floor and corresponds with the coccygeal plexus of nerves. In men it lies in the perineum, between the urinary and excretory openings. In women it is situated inside the posterior surface of the cervix.

This chakra relates to our feelings and perceptions and the bodily mechanisms associated with our survival, and explains the fear some grievers have with regard to their ability to continue simply going on living after a loss. In fact, even when we are actually safe and secure there can be underlying thoughts and emotions that turn on the fight-or-flight response, which produces an increased heart rate and sweaty palms. Because this is a basic "survival mode" reaction typical of human beings, it can be interpreted as a first chakra emanation, symbolizing our primary instinct for survival, our clinging to existence while fearing natural processes like death.

We recognize how attachment to pleasure-giving sensory objects and aversion toward external sources of displeasure become hardwired. When faced with grief, we can understand how oftentimes the griever wishes to join the deceased, as if his or her very survival were linked to the continuity of the bond. Because grief can seduce us to mistakenly identify the loss of a loved one as a threat to our existence, the result can be a natural inclination to merge with the deceased.

Because of its connection with the material world, we also see in this chakra the difficulty grievers typically experience in performing the usual tasks that ensure physical life. The fatigue that many people feel during grief is also typical of an imbalance in this center. This chakra is a potent source of all our earthly desires, and the fear, greed, and possessiveness we might feel when grieving are associated with it. An example could be wishing to hold on to a deceased's treasured objects or possessions.

Additionally, because the first chakra is associated with the sense of smell, the common occurrence of grievers being reminded suddenly of the deceased based on encountering a smell associated with that person can be seen as emanating from this chakra.

SACRAL CHAKRA: THE BIRTHPLACE OF DESIRE

The second chakra (*swadhisthana*) is found at the base of the spine. It relates to the sacral plexus of nerves and symbolizes the unconscious. It is also related to our overall emotional awareness and ability to experience our feelings. Strongly connected to the sexual organs and their products, desires and cravings take on definite form and direction in this chakra. This chakra is also associated with movement, especially emotional types of movement. In terms of grief, the involvement of this chakra can manifest as a lack of sexual desire or, conversely, a strengthening of sexual appetite. The difficulty some experience in accessing intimacy or being social with others is a typical characteristic of a disturbed second chakra. The associated sense with this chakra is taste. Sometimes there is a certain taste some grievers notice along with other, more typical symptoms such as dry mouth and disruptions of normal eating habits.

NAVAL CHAKRA: WILLPOWER MADE MANIFEST

The third chakra (*manipura*) sits along the spinal column directly behind the navel. It corresponds to the solar plexus and physiologically relates to digestion, assimilation, and temperature regulation in the body. This chakra represents an important step in the evolution of consciousness because it connects our willpower with our desires, promoting manifestation on the physical plane. The difficulty in making decisions felt by many grievers is an involvement of the third chakra. We become confused as to what course of action is best because our willpower is so profoundly compromised. We sometimes resort to taking no action at all, lacking the motivation needed to confront the fear of the changes we are facing.

Some individuals throw themselves into work. Others place a heightened emphasis on an exuberant social life after loss to keep away from the painful lack of familiarity with the new unchartered reality. The literal translation of *manipura* is "city of jewels," and it refers to the precious gems of action lying dormant in this center, waiting to be unearthed by the power of our conscious intention. The associated sense for this chakra is sight, and I believe it can explain common experiences some bereaved have of not seeing things that are in plain sight—for example, searching frantically for house keys, only to find them in the appropriate place just a few minutes later; or not seeing the exit sign on the freeway, even though it is the same exit a griever has taken for the past five years when returning home. Even "seeing" the deceased within the midst of a crowd on a busy street could be related to the third chakra.

HEART CHAKRA: THE REFUGE OF LOVE

The fourth chakra (*anahata*) lies in the vertebral column behind the base of the heart at the level of the depression in the sternum. It relates to the cardiac plexus of nerves, which influences the functioning of the heart and lungs. These are two key areas that are often affected by grief, manifesting as disruptions of both cardiac and breathing rhythms. The heart chakra corresponds to the thymus gland, which relates to immune function. During bereavement it is common to experience an exacerbation of preexisting health conditions or an increased risk for sickness due to immune system depression. This chakra is the quintessential blending of matter and Spirit, the evolutionary oasis on our path toward spiritual fulfillment. It is where emotional bonding and attachment are developed. As the seat of human love, it also relates to the power of love as a healing force.

The sense associated with *anahata* is touch. In grief, this sense is important because through touch we fully experience the absence of that which we have lost. Just think of the need many individuals feel for touch after spousal loss. Imagine how liberating a hug can feel to facilitate the powerful release of pent-up emotion.

THROAT CHAKRA: THE POWER OF SOUND

The fifth chakra (*vishuddhi*) lies at the level of the throat pit in the vertebral column. This chakra corresponds to the cervical plexus of nerves and relates to the thyroid gland and also certain systems of articulation, the upper palate, and the epiglottis. The thyroid's involvement is key in grief: the disturbance of the production of adrenaline can be the source of feelings of depletion, as well as weight gain or loss that cannot be directly attributable to changes in eating habits. This center can also be the source for some of the hormonal imbalances and mood swings experienced when grieving.

Vishuddhi chakra is known as the purification center, where the powers of communication lie. It deals symbolically with sound and vibration. Often, those grieving have difficulty talking about their grief or articulating their feelings about a loss. The overwhelming need for some grieving individuals to have their stories heard is another indication of this chakra's involvement. Because the associated sense with this chakra is hearing, we can understand the importance of voicing painful as well as joyful memories in the midst of loss. Fifth-chakra disturbances can also result in sore throats and pain in the neck and shoulders—areas very commonly affected by grief. The sensation of feeling choked can be associated with this chakra as well.

THIRD-EYE CHAKRA: WISDOM FOUND WITHIN

The sixth chakra (*ajna*) lies in the midline of the brain directly above the spinal column and corresponds with the pineal gland. This chakra controls the muscles and the onset of sexual activity in humans. It has control over all the functions of the body. It is the chakra of pure mind, representing a higher level of awareness. It is usually called the "third eye," and it is said that whereas the two physical eyes look outward, the third eye looks inward. In that sense it reveals the intuitive knowledge independent from the information supplied by the senses.

Ajna is the witnessing center where one becomes the detached observer of all events, including those within the body and the mind. Sleep disorders are a typical involvement of this chakra because of its relationship to the pineal gland and its main biochemical product, melatonin. Because of its connection with inner vision, we might experience broader issues related to our perception, finding difficulty in seeing the road ahead. Other common symptoms include coordination problems, such as accidentally bumping into the furniture.

On a positive note, this chakra serves as a reminder that it is by looking within that we find the source of all the feelings and thoughts that come up during the upheaval created by loss. By witnessing the endless fluctuations and changes within our own minds, we can approach stillness. In essence, while our minds struggle to understand our losses, our Spirits know and are ready to accept them as a part of the normal cycle of life and existence. The source of the knowledge that we can apply to process grief comes from our connection with the intuitive wisdom the Spirit has rather than the acquired knowledge of the dualistic mind. It is because of this dualistic aspect of the mind, which is unable to recognize the night if it does not know the day, that we cling to the permanence of things, attempting to ensure the continuance of the treasured connections. The mind struggles to understand that even though a loved one may be absent, he or she is still present and interwoven in the fabric of our identity.

CROWN CHAKRA: WITNESS TO A GREATER REALITY

The seventh chakra (*sahasrara*) is the culmination of the kundalini's energetic pathway, seen as the seat of higher awareness. It is situated at the top of the head and is physically correlated to the pituitary gland, called the "command center," which regulates the entire endocrine system. On a symbolic level, it is in this chakra where the dual mind is transcended and we enter into perfect conscious harmony with the oneness of the universe. When this chakra is out of balance during bereavement it results in depression, alienation, and confusion. This chakra also relates to the challenges that grief imposes on one's own spiritual beliefs.

Body Armor: A Different Take on the Chakras

The chakra system identifies specific locations in the body and relates them with different types of emotions. Wilhelm Reich, the famous Austrian psycho-analyst, came up with a similar notion when he described his concept of "body armor;" he analyzed how mental conflicts are expressed in the body, often through muscular or nervous tension, and how this mechanism could be intended to protect the consciousness from accessing psychic content associated with these areas (1949).

Essentially, Reich's view is that we shield ourselves with the stiff armor of mus-cular tension and associated body language to avoid experiencing negative feel-ings. The fields of psychosomatic medicine and somatic psychotherapy have further deepened the study of these mechanisms and found revealing correlates between disease processes and what an individual is going through in his or her emotional and psychic life. For example, when an individual is dealing with boundary issues he or she might develop a skin condition. When someone finds it intolerable to examine one's reality, eye problems might develop. Of course, nothing is quite as simple as the examples given, yet the relationship between our minds and our bodies is undeniable.

When considering the wide variety of symptoms found in grief, it becomes evident that grief affects the whole being. Understanding the significance of the chakras in our physical bodies and how they relate to our overall experience is key in our thinking about grief when practicing. By learning the different roles that the chakras play in our bodies and how they affect us emotionally, the effects of our yoga practice are deepened. Exploring our knowledge of the chakra system leads to an efficient and helpful way to understand the mind-body connection and its relationship to the varying symptoms of grief.

The Heart Chakra: A Starting Point for Grief

Although all chakras are involved during the grieving process, the heart chakra is the primary one when talking about grief. Because emotional bonding develops there, *anahata* is an essential chakra to address when building a yoga practice for addressing the symptoms and considering the nature of the grieving process. It is the bridge between the lower chakras and the higher ones. In the words of John Selby, "[B]elow the heart chakra, lies the world of matter, of survival and procreation, of manipulation and mastery over the physical realms of life. Above lies the world of Spirit, of pure thought and intuition, of interpersonal communication and, ultimately, universal unity and transcendence. The heart chakra, in its most basic sense, is the marriage of matter and spirit, of concrete and abstract, of knowledge and wisdom, of earth and heaven" (1992, 147). It represents a specifically human kind of evolution, the growth of humanity out of depths of lower orders and emotions.

As the seat of love, this chakra is where our true challenge lies: when loss occurs, we must go through the difficult transition from "loving in presence" to "loving in absence." We can skillfully ask ourselves about the loss we are facing: Is our grief a consequence of pure love or pure attachment? It may be interesting to notice the overlapping of these closely related emotions, but according to yoga there is indeed a difference. As it is said in yoga, "Love is what's left after you've let go of everything you love." In this sense, attachment can be seen practically as the opposite of love, a concept that manifests in such phrases as "If you love something, let it go."

Yoga's quest for unconditional love also pertains to the idea that loving with the condition of presence is not real love. "I love you as long as you are around" is a rather limiting concept, one that does not honor the expansiveness of love. It is yet another example of the dualistic mind that validates reality based on physical presence. What we cannot see, what we cannot touch, we tend to treat as nonexistent. To accept that love continues despite the absence of our attachment, we must transcend dualistic thinking and embrace the inevitability of change.

Practicing yoga helps us to better understand this duality of love and attachment. By developing a deeper awareness of and working on our heart chakra and the physical sensations and functions associated with it, an individual can experience enlightening expansion resulting in profound healing. We gain the ability to synthesize our physical, mental, and spiritual awareness into a practice that acknowledges both the relocation of the deceased and one's own continued presence on this plane of existence. What better way to honor a lost loved one?

Grief's Challenge to Spirituality

"Not yet settled in a permanent home, / the soul takes temporary shelter in a body," says Kural 340 (Subramuniyaswami 1999, 136). Ultimately, the difference between traditional psychotherapy's treatment of the griever and the yogic view is the special attention yoga gives to the Spirit. The solution for all causes of suffering offered in *The Yoga Sutras of Patanjali* is to reduce them to their source and deal with the resistance of the mind through meditation (Satyananda 1976). Some of the spiritual symptoms associated with grief can be seen in the following table:

SPIRITUAL SYMPTOMS OF GRIEF

- Feeling angry at God

- Asking questions about God, like: Why would God allow this?

- Asking questions about death and the deceased, such as: Where is she now? Is he okay? Can she see me? Will I see him again? What will happen when I die?

- Sensing the deceased's presence

- Hearing, smelling, or seeing the deceased

- Having death affirm or challenge beliefs

- Experiencing awe, wonder, mystery

- Reflecting on personal finitude

- Feeling the need to continue a relationship with the deceased

Table 5: Spiritual symptoms of grief

For some grievers loss causes a split from spirituality. Doubts surface about how life can continue in any meaningful way after someone dies. God's goodness is questioned when a child is killed. People often feel anger toward God when the loss they are going through seems senseless or unfair. For others, a similar loss can actually be a creative spark to one's individual spiritual journey, igniting a flame that yearns to connect with their untapped Spirit. Inquiry might result in finding new answers or in discarding the old ones.

Especially in the case of death, the losses we witness force us to face our own mortality. We analyze and question the nature of the relationship we have with our own Spirit. Impermanence as we know it forces us to question our beliefs, to inquire about the meaning of life, and to wonder about the unknown. Yoga draws inspiration from this type of self-inquiry. If in fact, as yoga teaches us, we have everything we need for a good life, then going within seems the right direction to take. Searching for the Spirit within then becomes a refuge, a valid place for understanding and creating meaning out of loss.

Love Beyond Attachment

Grief and suffering are intrinsically intertwined. Therefore yoga, as a spiritual discipline, is a natural fit as a useful system to address grief. Grief's relationship to attachment depicts the normal reaction to one of the five essential causes of suffering as stated by the sage Patanjali, establishing how love is different from, almost opposite to, attachment. Placed emotionally and physically in our heart chakra, love is the positive expression of the chakra, and attachment is the negative one.

In the Western view, attachment equals love and is almost a precondition for survival. Based on this, leaders in the field of grief work find that one of the goals of grief counseling and therapy is to develop new, healthier attachments. According to the teachings of yoga, this course of action leads to more suffering and actually undermines the transformative potential of our own grieving process. By accepting the ultimate truths that the universe is based on, and by relying on the impermanence of our objects of attachment, we can develop true and enduring love that transcends the limitations of the physical, placing love beyond attachment. Only then do we get in touch with our true essence—only then, rather than ending, our journey begins...

"The soul's attachment to the body is like that of a fledgling,
which forsakes its empty shell and flies away."

—Kural 338 (Subramuniyaswami 1999, 136)

Any valid practical model destined to help those who are grieving must include the spiritual challenges that grief presents. It must also deal with the ways in which the body expresses grief and the mind acknowledges the resulting suffering.

The following chapter demonstrates my contribution to assist grieving individuals with the complexities that grief entails. Out of necessity, we begin the journey of practice by meeting any difficulties with the forces of will. The results of the practice itself, and the wisdom one receives from this transformative endeavor, will both amaze and inspire you.

CHAPTER 3

How the Yoga for Grief Relief Practice Works

Regardless of which worldview—Western or Eastern—suits you best, it is important to remember that you must meet yourself where you are. In this chapter I offer insights related to the purpose of each category of exercises in relation to grief so that you can better understand how to address your needs. Before that begins, let's take a look at an important principle that applies to yoga in general: *The tool is never as important as the one who is wielding it.*

A piece of information, an exercise, or a technique is only useful if the operator is cautious, respectful, capable, and conscious. Whether you prefer the psychology-based approach of the Western model or the more spiritual understanding of Eastern philosophy, what's most important is to identify what you want to do with your grief by practicing yoga. The tools that you are about to receive will help aid you in your pursuit.

Here is a metaphor that may help you to understand the power of awareness located within yourself as you begin the practice: *The blacksmith can always forge himself a new hammer, but the hammer cannot make itself a new blacksmith.* In other words, you will see that the process of reidentification sprouts from the sorrowful seeds that lie amid your own grief.

As you start to move through the pain of loss, ask yourself how you will approach and engage in the yoga practice. What would you like to accomplish with it? As you incorporate various techniques to help cope with different symptoms encountered in your grief, you will notice changes in your body, mind, and emotions. Your experience each time you practice may be uniquely distinct, changing depending on the day, your mood, your physical state, or your life circumstances. Sometimes doing the same yoga technique in the morning instead of in the evening might reveal distinct information and produce very different effects on the practitioner. As you read this chapter, keep in mind that the intention of the practice is to contact that part of yourself that knows no loss. Some call it the observer, the higher self, or the true witness of all your experiences.

How This Practice Was Born

When I originally created this practice for transforming grief, a suitable sequence of techniques—the best possible information to serve grieving individuals—came pouring from within me with uncanny ease. I can only refer to this experience as an act of pure yogic inspiration. For years, I felt shy about sharing the way in which this practice came to life. Despite my strong sense of its therapeutic effectiveness, I feared people would underestimate the value of the sequence because it had not required months of struggle, elaborate study, or demanding intellectual focus. Experiencing this spontaneous reception of accurate and appropriate information produced in the depth of my being gave me humility and awe. Even personally knowing the magic of yoga, I still felt awkward about the ease with which this perfectly applicable *sadhana* showed itself, unveiling to me the tools to work with the bereaved.

Since that extraordinary moment back in 1994, I have personally witnessed the power of Yoga for Grief Relief at work. Whether in clinical or informal settings, group or private sessions, professional trainings or personal retreats, the transformational power of this *sadhana* continues to amaze me.

Incidentally, it was much later that I was able to identify that precious missing element in my awareness: yoga is within each one of us already. This knowledge often manifests as intuition that influences our creativity and all aspects of our lives. Initially my insights about the body's inherent involvement in the grieving process came from my own experience. I witnessed how my body expressed what my mind could not accept regarding the death of my beloved mother.

When she died I was a young man adamantly refusing to accept her death and the pain that resulted from it. Instead, I came up with multiple excuses for escaping my present reality, cleverly supporting my behavioral choices with thoughts that seemed to work. I told myself that my mom did not bring me up to be a sad creature mourning her death in every corner of our house. So I busied myself with studying and distracted myself with trips to the beach; I looked for excitement, dancing all night long, drinking and having a blast.

Two years after her death, the denial of the impact and the tearing of my heart manifested physically as a bone spur right in the center of my chest where one of my ribs meets the breastbone. It resembled calcifications that are produced internally after a fracture, orchestrated by the body to strengthen the skeletal system. Yes, I had a broken heart, and my body showed that to me.

When the Yoga for Grief Relief practice assumed its full form, it was embraced by practitioners as a useful set of tools affirming the effectiveness and perfection of engaging ancient yoga to address the various symptoms of modern-day grief. As I carefully built the Yoga for Grief Relief program, I first included exercises that I thought would take care of the more obvious bodily effects of grief. Next, I addressed the problem of perceptions of the bereaved mind in order to effect change in the neuroendocrine system. Finally, I sought to help people change their perception of the loss and redefine themselves based on a newfound self-awareness.

The Active Principles of the Practice

Yoga offers techniques to enhance our awareness of the inherent, vibrant unity among body, mind, and spirit. For the body, yoga offers *asanas*, or physical movements, that improve vital functions and enhance emotional awareness. For the mind, yoga uses *pranayama*, or breath work. Because the quality and rhythm of our breathing changes as we experience different thoughts and emotions, actively working with our breathing patterns can be a useful way to address the mental symptoms encountered in grief. Finally, yoga offers meditation to address the Spirit, since once the body is still and the mind entertained, that which is neither mind nor body can more fully manifest.

The yoga system is precise in how it prescribes exercises for specific symptoms much like Western medicine does, yet it is unique in acknowledging that each exercise addresses the full being. The six significant categories that help us to move through the grieving process are breath work, body movements, cleansing techniques, relaxation, mind reprogramming, and meditation.

Pranayama: Introducing Life Control Through Breath Work

Pranayama involves working directly with our most abundant life-bestowing energy: our breath (*prana*). These exercises restore our sense of control by connecting us to our innermost vitality, which easily falls out of balance after loss. Consciously working with our breath helps to reestablish balance and cope with the fearsome loss of control that grief often presents. It also helps us to acquaint ourselves with our minds more intimately, to observe the ways in which we process our emotions. Based on this observation, we can decide which tools we need to use to activate our energy when feeling depleted, or to relax and feel calm when feeling anxious.

Because breathing is automatic and normally performed unconsciously, working consciously with the breath helps us to bridge the gap between conscious and unconscious. Each time we engage the breath this way we help unite the intentional conscious mind and the more hidden unconscious mind, allowing us to focus on those aspects that remain in the shadowy corners of our awareness.

It is impossible to change that which we don't know or acknowledge. We need to recognize the existence of something before we can transform it. It is through our breath awareness that we anchor our authentic experience, bringing attention to life in the present moment. Our challenge is acknowledging the actual moment as is rather than what we think about it; the intention is to actually experience and view the concrete reality of the moment.

In Uruguay, where I was born, there is a popular saying: "A life is to write a book, to plant a tree, and to bring up a child." My spiritual master, Maharaji Prem Pal Singh Rawat, gives it a beautiful twist, saying, "Life is one breath in and one breath out, no more, no less. So actually writing a book, planting a tree, or bringing up a child are 'stories' of life" (1990). Giving presence to our breath, we give presence to our life as well.

The tedious nature of the bereavement process demands, or at least requests, patience and awareness, something conscious breathing develops. After all, it is not possible to take the next breath before the present one is complete: this is the only way in which life can happen, just one breath at a time.

Asana: Tools for Transforming the Body

Specific physical poses alter the symptoms of grief by addressing pain, lack of energy, and various structural malformations our bodies can contort into, such as hunched backs or caved-in chests. These tools for somatic transformation can be put into practice to promote movement of the physical and psychic contents in the body. Essentially, any symptom, whether psychological or physical, indicates a blockage of energy resulting in the disruption of the natural balance of our health. By promoting the movement of energy, we allow the life force to flow to those places in the body that need it the most. We also bring the latent contents of our minds to the surface of consciousness, making them available to witness, explore, and ultimately transform.

Our bodies are profoundly involved in the grieving process and infinitely wiser than our minds. Tapping into the body's wisdom through movement, while monitoring our intensified sensations and feelings, gives us a much-needed awareness of the connection of body and mind. Intentionally engaging our body in these practices is essential for our continued optimal health and well-being.

Establishing the connection mentally and physically allows the mind to use the body as an anchor during times of unrest.

When faced with an experience that we perceive as threatening, we tend to shield ourselves with emotional armor built from previous pain and suffering. Habitually cutting off the flow of our life force to avoid contact with unpleasant feelings literally prevents us from processing the pain of our emotions. Like a house of cards built on illusion, this charade depletes our resources and distracts us from the task of working with our authentic feelings.

Performing these *asanas* challenges the holdings of the body's armor (see "Body Armor: A Different Take on the Chakras," in chapter 2) and helps the natural energy hubs (chakras) connect, enhancing the continuous flow of consciousness. By stirring up the emotional and psychic contents held in the muscle memory, we can connect with our story through our body's display of both strength and weakness.

As you will find, many of the *asanas* presented here support the body's vigorous challenge to face the symptoms of grief. Yogic action is greatly valued and especially effective in transforming grief. Among the many other benefits yoga offers, choosing specific postures helps the body release some of the unwanted grief-induced chemicals present in the blood stream.

Shatkarma: A Cleansing Technique for the Mind

Shatkarma is a group of yogic cleansing techniques used to release emotions, thoughts, or physical experiences trapped in the body-mind. This process can be likened to cleaning the surface of a crystal. First it allows us to deal with the grime, then it addresses what lies below, and finally it encounters the pristine clarity of the crystal undisturbed by what clouded it.

In the particular case of dealing with grief, belief systems, worldviews, and preexisting mental programming usually cloud our ability to perceive our grief as normal. The toxic byproducts of stress, the debilitating action on the immune system, and the neurologically induced negative anticipatory thinking can and must be transformed so we can start to feel better and diligently and purposefully access the hidden gem found within grief.

Relaxation: Combating Stress

Relaxing practices such as *anga shaithilya*, or self-relaxation, are vital for diminishing stress levels that are usually heightened during grief. Adjusting to our new, undefined reality often involves learning new coping skills. For some of us, that alone can increase stress. Relaxation is a potent normalizer and antidote to deal with the resulting symptoms of both somatically expressed stress and mental anguish. *Anga shaithilya* also helps regulate disturbed vital functions such as breathing and cardiac rhythms, sleep cycles, and eating habits. Relaxation is also fundamental in helping the body achieve homeostasis, balancing blood-pressure levels, and resetting the overall endocrine system, which, in turn, helps to reduce our dramatic mood swings and general state of irritability.

Sankalpa: Resetting the Mind

One of the most effective mental reprogramming techniques yoga possesses is *Sankalpa*, the powerful yogic principle referred to as "Resolve." Setting our intention or saying a prayer, often out loud, can help reset the brain and focus the mind. The application for grief in particular helps address the scattered and shattered linear thinking that is so characteristic of grief. By focusing the mind and identifying the present situation, grieving individuals can clarify what specific changes they intend to accomplish. This tool is simply called Resolve and it surely "resolves!" This practice engages our full presence, indicating that one is resolved to take the next step. Resolve combats negative anticipatory thinking that stems from grief-induced disturbances of the limbic system. It accomplishes this by formulating intentions only in the present tense, producing positive mental alignment and offering a powerful antidote for fear-based ruminations.

Meditation: The Chief Technique to Address the Spirit

Many people think meditation involves stopping the mind. Due to this erroneous misconception, many frustrated and confused seekers choose to totally discard meditation. In truth, the attempt to stop the mind is futile since it contradicts the mind's inherent functioning, which constantly shifts from the past to the future, from the real to the fantasized. Rather than attempting to stop the mind, meditation offers the ever-changing mind a limited range of change—for example, going from chanting one om to another, or moving from one repetition of the Rosary to another one. This, in turn, comfortably distracts the mind due to a natural feature of the brain that masks permanent stimuli.

To better understand this masking feature, imagine someone who moves to a new home in front of railroad tracks and hears each and every passing train. A few months later, while entertaining at home, a dinner guest expresses profound concern about the intense noise: "Wow, these trains must drive you crazy!" The host queries unthinkingly, "What trains?"

How the Practice Functions as a Whole

The *sadhana* that I've developed follows its own inherent rhythm, leading us through progressive steps for transforming grief. First it helps us prepare to be present for the full palette of our feelings, then it promotes the proper flow of life force, creating optimal conditions for healing. Next it stirs the emotional heart, deepening our connection with our emotions, and then it provides an outlet for the ones we want to release. Subsequently, it offers some control over the emotional roller coaster of grief so that balance can then be achieved. Through relaxation, the deep release of internal and external stressors follows, readying the mind to access new programming. We then have a more direct, unobstructed pathway to the depth of our Spirit for creatively redefining our new identity.

Overcoming Barriers to Practice

The *sadhana* presented in this book is a practice. Therefore it requires your commitment to practice for you to reap the desired benefits. This may seem obvious to you, yet that is not so for many people. Some hope that by simply reading this material their symptoms will spontaneously abate. Others, although encouraged by the results seen after just a few initial rounds, simply will stop practice because they do not have the will or strength within to continue. Some report that they don't practice because of lack of appropriate support; others because they are waiting for the most ideal conditions that never seem to show up. All of these are excuses that can and must be resolved.

Success in yoga and the ability to manifest the best possible life is based on two core principles: practice and nonattachment. Working on nonattachment is by far more difficult than working on establishing a practice. Especially during excruciatingly difficult moments of bereavement, the grieving mind may well resist talking about or confronting the concept of nonattachment.

As stated in chapter 1, we only grieve the loss of that which we are attached to. This statement depicts exactly how grief and attachment are intrinsically intertwined.

Each part of the *sadhana* serves the overall goal of transforming the complex experience of grief by promoting body, mind, and spirit integration and rejuvenation.

To accommodate the emotional waves and inherent fluctuations in the bereavement process, I suggest maintaining an attitude of detachment toward the immediate results of practice. Some days your practice will be intense; on others it may be milder. Some days you will feel content after practicing; other days your practice might take you to places that feel less than satisfying. The deeper benefits will come as a result of establishing a regular practice. Keep in mind that in the best-case scenario, a serious, dedicated practice can actually lead one to nonattachment.

In the following chapter, I will demonstrate how to do the practices themselves, how each practice helps us, and how to establish the best logistics to ensure a successful practice.

CHAPTER 4

What You Can Do: The Yoga Practice

This chapter features the *sadhana*, a sequence of exercises presented in a simple way and a specific order best suited to aid in your grieving process. The previous chapter shared information explaining the general effects of each group of exercises. This chapter explains how each technique specifically addresses grief and how to practice each one by following step-by-step instructions. The chapter that follows this one will help you discern how and when to use the exercises and, if need be, how to adapt them according to your personal abilities and needs. You may benefit from familiarizing yourself with both chapters as you embark on your practice, alternating between the two while learning the techniques and planning how to integrate them into your life.

Here is an at-a-glance list of the *sadhana* exercises (along with their Sanskrit names) in the order I propose they be practiced in:

Yoga for Grief Relief *Sadhana*

Pranayama

    Complete Breathing (*Mahat Yoga Pranayama*)

Asana

Energy Flow Series (*Pawanmuktasana* 1)

Windmill (*Vayu Chakram Asana*)

Attitude of Discharging (*Utthita Lolasana*)

Shatkarma

Concentrated Gazing (*Tratak*)

Pranayama

Alternate-Nostril Breathing (*Nadi Shodhana Pranayama*)

Relax

Self-Relaxation Technique (*Anga Shaithilya*)

Mental Reprogramming

Resolve (*Sankalpa*)

Meditation

Breath Meditation

Accepting Life Fully

"Life is one breath in and one breath out..."

—Prem Pal Singh Rawat

Practicing Complete Breathing allows you to get in touch with the quintessential movement in your life: one breath in and one breath out. During bereavement the mind is confused in its attempt to grasp a new reality, and tends to ruminate on the past or anticipate a negative future. Since neither of these tendencies allow you to inhabit the present—the only place to really be—it is important to bring awareness to what life is really like in the moment. This exercise calms the mind while the body benefits from receiving a proper intake of oxygen, which helps to alleviate the shortness of breath commonly present when grieving.

Complete Breathing (*Mahat Yoga Pranayama*)

Prior to actually practicing Complete Breathing, let's take a look at a preparatory exercise that will help you better identify the three parts involved in the technique.

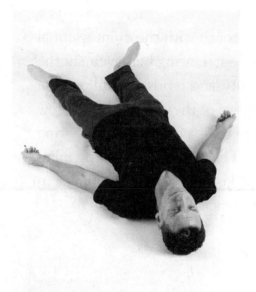

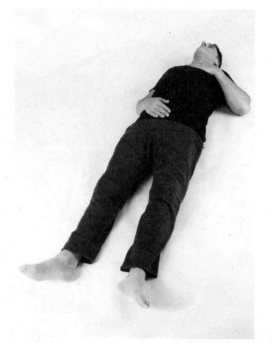

Preparation for Complete Breathing

1. Lie on your back, find a comfortable position, and place your arms at your sides with palms facing up.

2. Connect with your breath and observe the breath's natural rhythm. Observe the involvement of your belly, ribs, and chest in your breath.

3. Bring your right hand to the lower belly, keeping the elbow on the floor. Bring the left hand onto your chest. Inhale, bringing air mostly to the belly. Exhale, softly contracting the belly. Continue to breathe this way for a few rounds. Note that at this time there should be no movement of your left hand or in the rib cage area. Witness the right hand moving up and down while the left remains still.

4. Now move both hands to the rib cage, placing the thumb at the back of the ribs close to the spine and your fingers in front. Make sure that the inner edge of the hands (thumb to the tip of the index finger) follows the curve of your ribs. Rest the tip of the index finger as close to the front part of the ribs as you can. Inhale, allowing the ribs to

expand. Exhale, allowing the ribs to come back toward the center of your body as they contract. Compress the ribs slightly toward the center of the body with your hands at the end of the exhalation. Continue to breathe this way for a few rounds. Note that the chest and belly should experience little movement at this time.

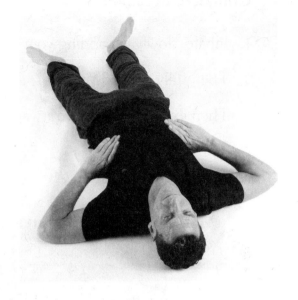

5. Place your hands back at your sides for a moment before bringing them to their previous position: left hand at the chest, right hand at the lower belly. Inhale, allowing the chest to fill up. Notice the collarbones moving toward the jawbone. Then exhale, allowing the chest to softly contract as it returns to the original position. Continue to breathe this way for a few rounds. At this time, there should be no movement of the belly, the right hand, or the rib cage area.

Now that each phase of breathing has been broken down for you, bring it together in sequence as Complete Breathing.

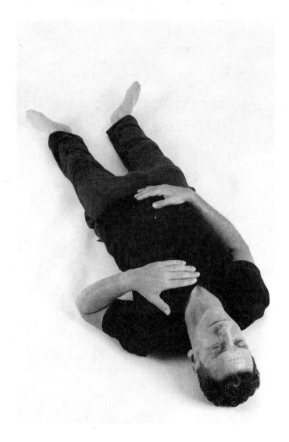

Complete Breathing

1. Inhale, slowly expanding your abdomen.

2. Then fully expand your ribs.

3. Then expand the chest outward and upward.

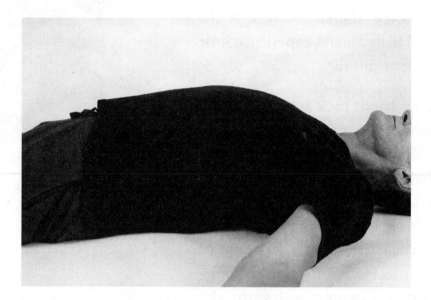

4. Exhale, relaxing first the abdomen, then the ribs, and then the chest, first downward and then inward.

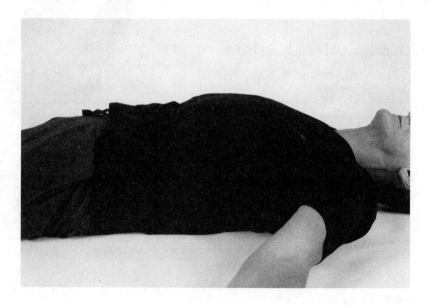

5. Practice continuous inhalations and exhalations. There may be a tendency to allow the belly to fall while bringing air into the chest. Do your best to keep the belly full during inhalation and as you continue to engage the remaining parts.

Suggested time: 5 minutes.

Benefits

- It maximizes your inhalations and exhalations.

- It helps you gain control of the breath, corrects altered breathing patterns, and increases oxygen intake.

- It brings awareness to the area where the main chakras are located, therefore enhancing conscious connection with related thoughts and sensations.

- It serves as a symbolic acceptance of the totality of the grieving process.

- It helps promote a psychological sensation of greater control over life.

Precautions

- The whole process should be one continuous movement.

- Each phase of breathing moves into the next without any obvious transition point.

- If experiencing lower back pain, place a cushion or other support under your knees.

Contraindications

- None.

On a psychosomatic level, by engaging your abdominal muscles during Complete Breathing you can connect with gut feelings such as anger, fear, or guilt. Raw feelings experienced by the heart often encounter resistance from the mind. There is a reason why many people refer to feeling anxious as having a knot in their stomach.

The intercostal muscles hold the ribs together and relate to safety. They are the muscles that help protect our precious vital organs. It is common to see the rib cage locked in defense with frightened and abused individuals. By tensing the intercostals, an individual attempts to re-create a sense of security that is being threatened. Asking yourself questions to identify the threat—"What is threatening me? How can I maintain a sense of security? What might I need to do?"—can skillfully elicit much-needed introspection. Allowing the rib cage to expand is symbolic of your intention to be flexible regarding safety.

The pectoral breath relates to emotions or your elaborated gut feelings. Most of us first filter our gut feelings through the parameters of what we consider safe, then transform them into complex emotions including other aspects related to our belief systems, intellectual considerations, learned defense mechanisms, and more.

"The way in which you breathe is a metaphor for the way in which you are living your life. Are you taking little sips of breath as though you don't have permission to take up much space on the planet?" asks Amy Weintraub (2004, 125). Your practice of Complete Breathing is symbolic of your commitment to a full breath and a full life. Therefore, you are able to truly inhabit the present and deal with the feelings that grief stirs up. You might not like these feelings, yet it is necessary to be present for them if the intention is to move through the grief process in a healthy way. By exhaling fully you are also committing to completely letting go of what no longer serves you—perhaps a good trade-off!

Some people know a different way of practicing this technique called Durga: using belly, ribs, and chest to inhale, but exhaling using chest first, then ribs, and belly last. I propose using belly, ribs, then chest for both inhalation and exhalation because it facilitates filling and also emptying the lungs most efficiently. Imagine one of those tubes of frosting with a metal tip used for decorating cakes. If you really want to empty it, you must first press the bottom, then the middle, and last the tip. The same applies to the lungs, which are basically two triangles with the base facing toward the bottom of the torso. The lungs empty most completely when lowering the belly first, then the ribs, then the chest. This action also allows for a stronger inhalation after each exhalation because nothing can be filled up completely if it has not been previously emptied.

After you have mastered the use of the three areas involved in this breath work, please practice Complete Breathing using your personal breathing rhythm. Practicing breathing in the way I've indicated can be symbolically used as a sign of your willingness to embrace the fullness of your grieving process. Once the breath is made conscious and its use enhanced by the practice of Complete Breathing, then we can attempt to control the flow of life force.

Unblocking the Flow of the Life Force

This *asana* series is a masterpiece of yoga—a true gem—though, perhaps due to its simplicity, deceptive power, and gentle efficiency, it is not always acknowledged as such. Unblocking the life force's flow is essential when attempting to regain health and promote change. The word *pawan* means "divine wind" and relates to the life force that comes with the breath; *mukta* means "release," and *asana* means "pose." Therefore, *pawanmuktasana* translates to poses that remove blockages that prevent the free flow of energy in both body and mind. This technique should be practiced from beginning to end without skipping any part.

Energy Flow Series (*Pawanmuktasana* 1)

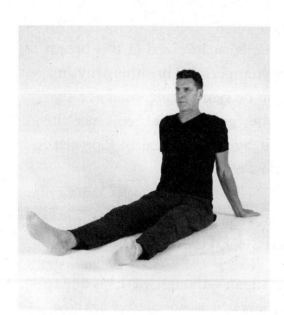

Sit with your legs straight and your hands behind your body, fingers pointing away from your toes.

Toe Bending

1. Bring awareness to your toes.

2. Now roll the toes forward, then back.

3. Keep your awareness on your toes.

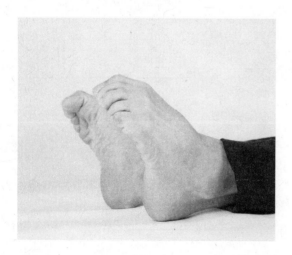

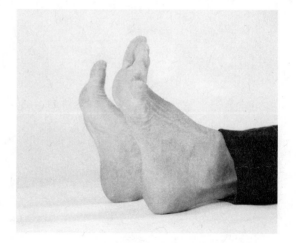

Ankle Bending

1. Separate your legs slightly so that when you perform ankle rotations your feet do not touch.

2. Bring awareness to your ankles.

3. Rotate your ankles in opposite directions, keeping the toes relaxed. Make as wide a rotation as you comfortably can.

4. Now reverse directions.

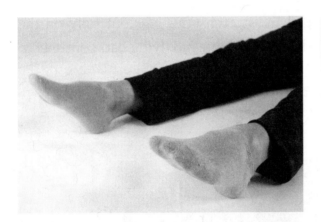
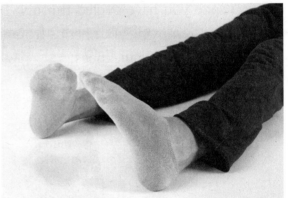
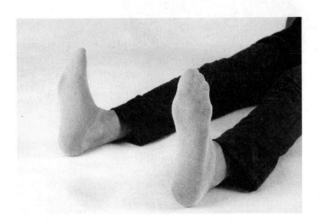
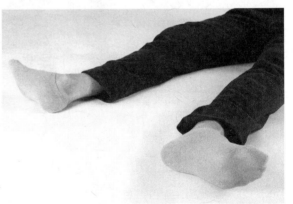

Knee Bending

1. Bring awareness to your knees.

2. Lie down on your back, with your hands under the sacrum, palms facing down, and the soles of your feet on the floor, knees bent.

3. Straighten your right leg up fully.

4. Let the calf fall, bending at the knee.

5. Now switch legs and repeat.

6. Once you have cycled through both legs, stretch your legs out fully on the floor, removing your hands from under the sacrum; and, lying flat, continue to be aware of your knees.

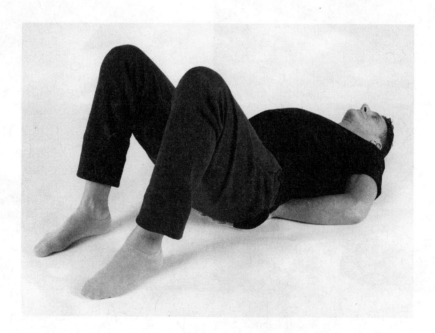

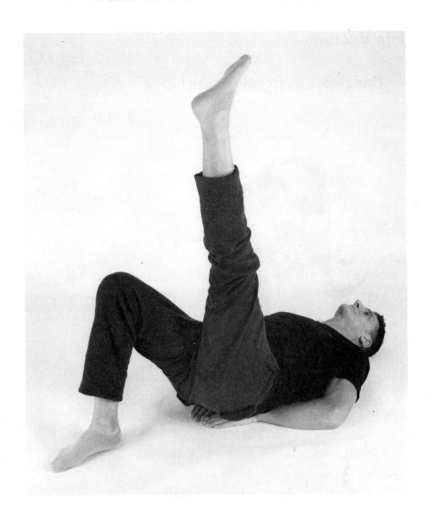

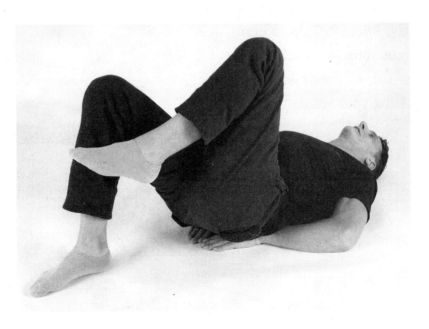

Hip Rotation

1. Bring your awareness to the hips.

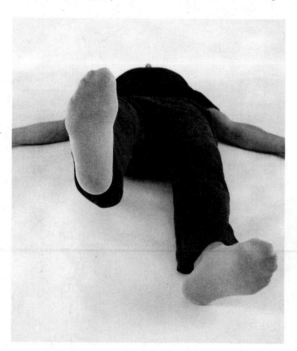

2. Lift the right leg slightly off the floor.

3. Cross the right leg low over the left leg toward your left arm, keeping the knee straight. Keep your gluteus muscles, back, and shoulders flat on the floor to avoid twisting your waist.

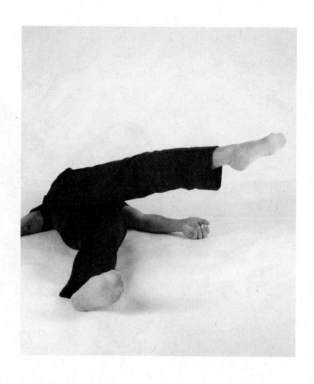

4. Bend the right knee, bringing it toward your face.

5. Open the right leg out to the right and straighten the knee.

6. Bring the right leg toward the left leg.

7. Continue with the rotation, making another large circle.

8. Repeat the cycle with the same leg but rotate in the opposite direction.

9. Repeat with the left leg.

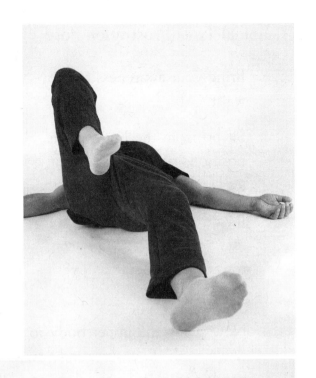

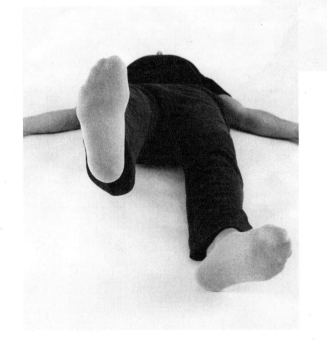

Spinal Twist Prostration Pose

1. Bring your awareness to the waist.

2. Sit up from the lying down position, and spread your legs apart.

3. Inhale and bend the body forward, bringing your arms toward your toes.

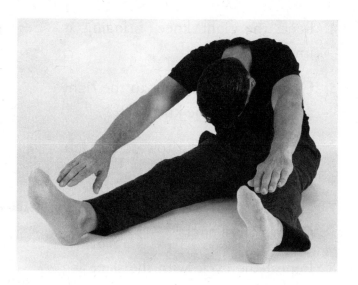

4. Now swing the upper body to the left and, on an exhale, bring your torso down to the floor, creating a twist at the waist. You should end up with your hands and chin on the floor and elbows up. Make sure you leave your right buttock as close to the floor as you can, while also bringing the left shoulder down toward the floor.

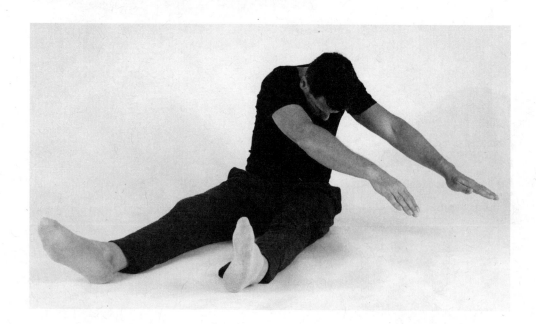

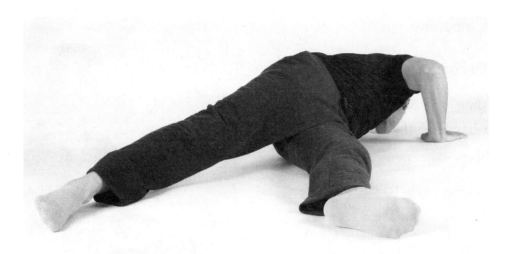

5. Now inhale and come up, swinging the upper body back toward your feet.

6. On an exhale, swing the body to the right side.

7. Repeat.

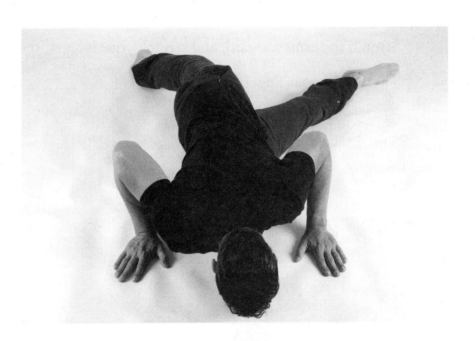

Be sure your chin rests where the back of your head would be if you were lying down.

Hand Clenching

1. Find a comfortable sitting position.

2. Keeping the spine straight, bring your hands to the knees, with palms facing up.

3. Bring awareness to your fingers.

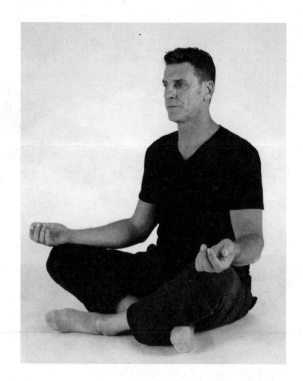

4. Stretch the arms forward, and stretch your fingers, spreading them apart.

5. Then bend your fingers in, creating two fists.

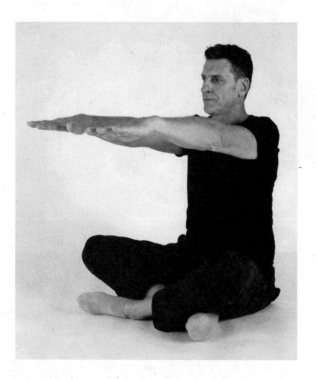

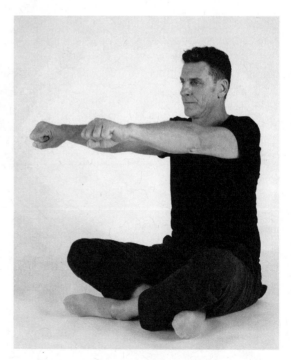

6. Uncurl your fingers and bring your hands back down to rest on your knees, keeping awareness on your fingers.

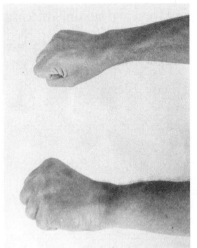
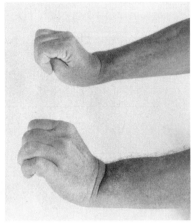
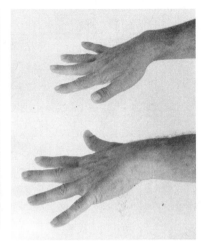

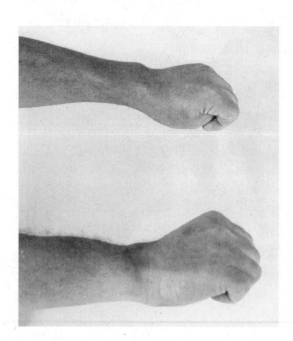

Wrist-Joint Rotation

1. Move awareness to your wrists.

2. Stretch the arms forward again, making two fists. Keep your thumbs inside the fists.

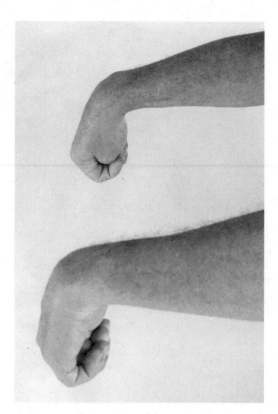

3. Keeping your hands in that position, bring them up, and rotate your wrists in opposite directions. Keep your arms parallel with the floor, and make sure to keep them straight, the forearms facing down, rotating only the wrists.

4. Now reverse the direction.

5. Bring your hands back to the knees, relax them, and remain with your awareness on the wrists.

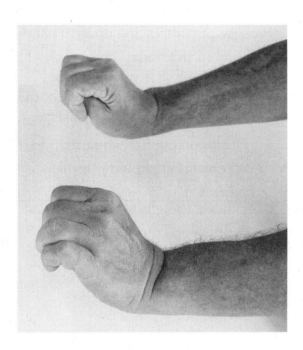

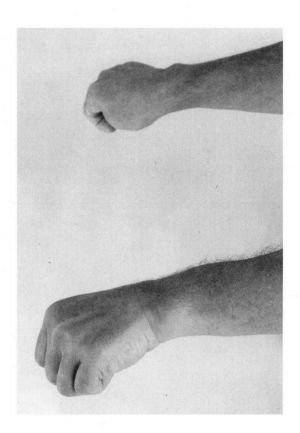

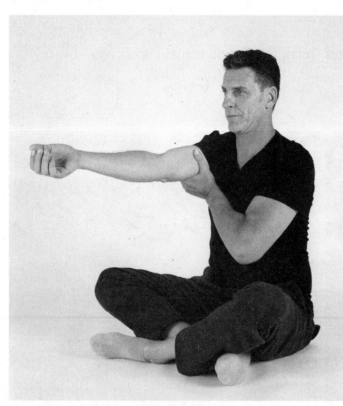

Elbow Bending

1. Bring your awareness to the elbows.

2. Stretch the right arm forward, with palm facing up, arm parallel to the floor.

3. Hold the right arm with the left hand at the bicep area, supporting the whole arm so it remains at shoulder level.

4. Bend the elbow, bringing your fingers to the shoulder.

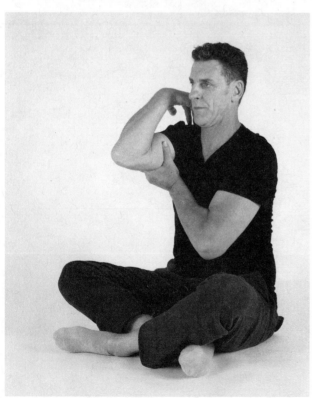

5. Now let the forearm fall forward, straightening your arm again, with the palm facing up.

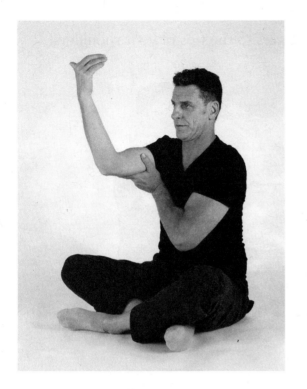 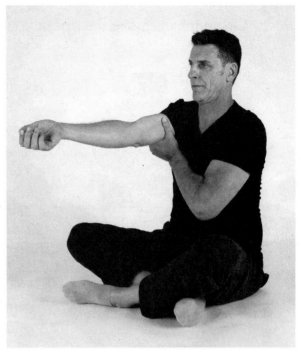

6. Change arms, and repeat.

7. Now bring your arms down, relaxing them and placing your hands at the knees.

8. Keep your awareness on the elbows.

Shoulder Socket Rotation

1. Bring awareness to your shoulders.

2. On an inhale, move the tips of your fingers to the tips of your shoulders.

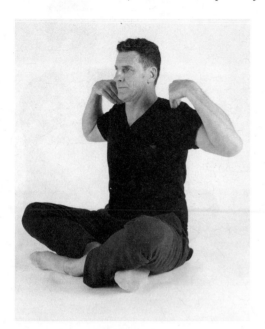 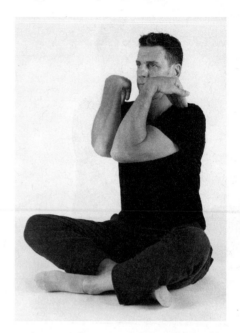

3. Exhale, placing the elbows together in front of your chest. Your elbows should touch.

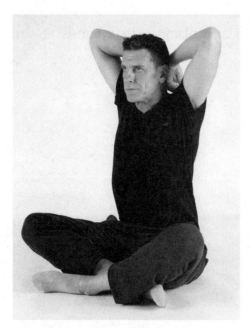 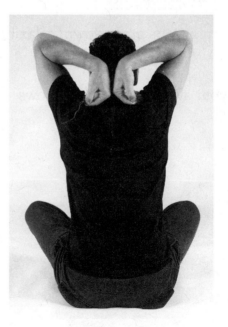

4. Inhale, bringing the elbows up, then back. Make sure the hands touch at the back of the neck.

5. Exhale, bringing the elbows down, then forward, completing the circle. Make sure to keep the neck relaxed.

6. Repeat the exercise with the elbows rotating in the opposite direction.

7. When done, bring your hands to rest on the knees, relaxing the shoulders.

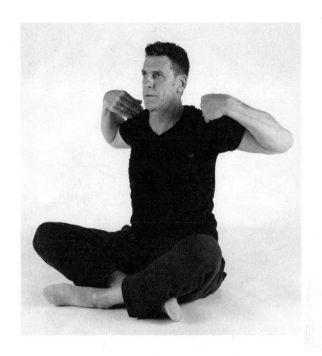

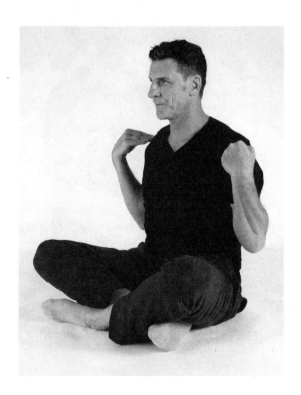

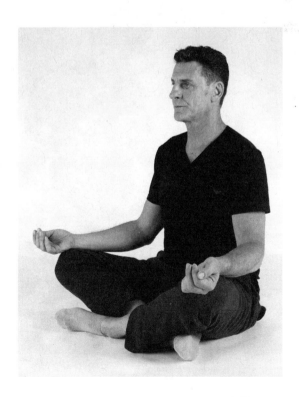

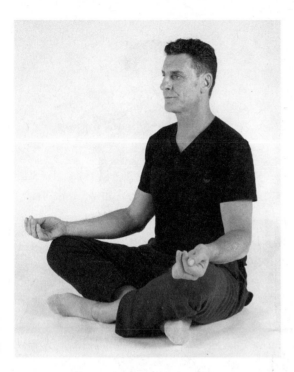

Neck Rotations

1. Bring awareness to your neck.

2. Let the head fall forward.

3. Now bring the head up, then let it roll back, opening the mouth slightly.

4. Repeat the motion.

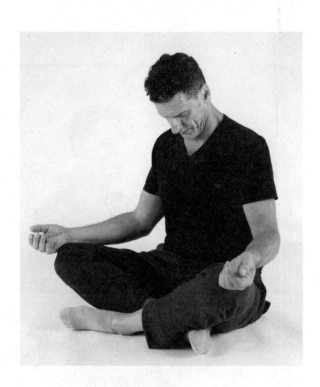

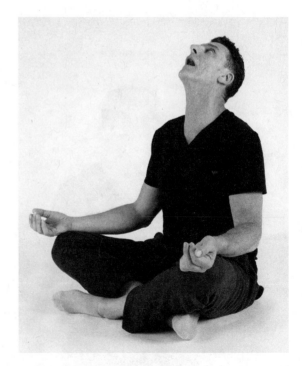

5. Now bring your head back straight to its original position and tilt it slightly to the right, bringing the right ear down toward the right shoulder.

6. Bring the head back up and tilt it to the left, bringing the left ear down toward the left shoulder. Don't turn your neck; only move the head.

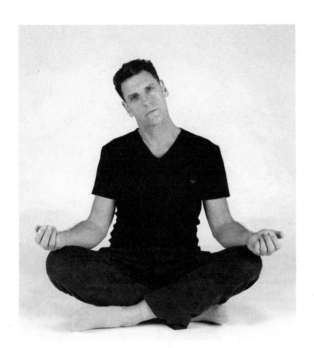 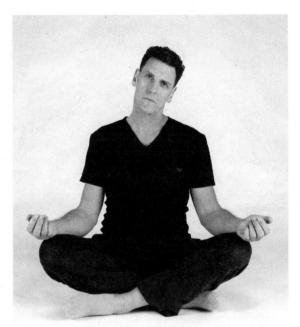

7. Now bring the chin down to your chest.

8. Bring the chin up and move it toward the right shoulder.

9. Then bring your chin up, pointing it toward the ceiling.

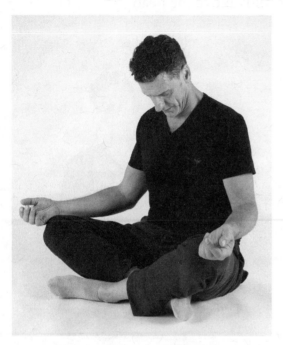

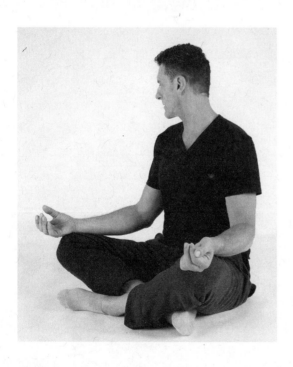

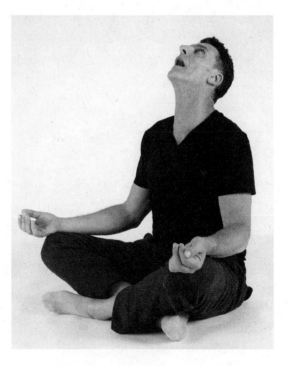

10. Now move your chin toward the left shoulder.

11. Then bring it down toward the chest.

12. Reverse directions. Remember to keep your shoulders and hands relaxed as you cycle through the movements. Keep your awareness on your neck.

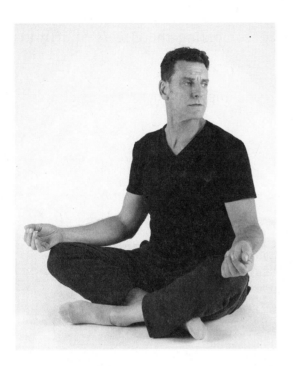
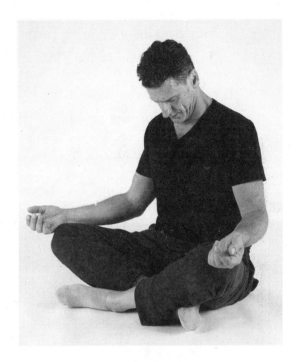

Suggested number of repetitions: no less than 3 times each movement.
Suggested time: 10 minutes.

Benefits

- It promotes the free flow of life force.

- It optimizes the conditions for healing.

- It stimulates proper lymphatic drainage.

- It improves proper joint functionality, combating the effects of arthritis and other degenerative illnesses.

- It relaxes the muscles of the body and the impulses that travel back to the brain, relaxing the mind.

- It tunes up the autonomic nerves.

- It balances hormonal functions.

- It improves vital organ functions.

- It improves the attentive faculty of the mind.

Precautions

- Stay focused on each body part prior to moving it, while moving it, and afterward as well.

- Be sensitive to pain associated with potential popping sounds when moving the hips. If the popping is not painful, you might continue.

- If momentarily unable to perform a movement, do not skip that joint or place. Rather, visualize the movement as fully as you are able to, then continue with the subsequent joint.

Contraindications

- This series needs to be modified if you have injuries or limitations in any particular joint involved.

- Those suffering from sciatica or lower back–related conditions should be sensitive to pain when performing those *asanas* that involve this area of the body.

- The neck exercises should not be performed fully by those suffering from high blood pressure or extreme cervical spondylosis.

As we free the energy in our body it flows from healthy places to compromised areas, promoting the flow of the life force, nourishing the body from within, and allowing it to heal. Grief is not an illness, although at times we certainly feel quite sick. Our bodies ache, yearning for the reestablishment of our well-being. As practice helps to restore order and proper overall functioning, we are more equipped to cope with grievous health disturbances.

Placing our awareness on each joint helps us gain deeper contact with ourselves, heightening our perception of sensations and feelings in the body.

Doing this offers the possibility of tapping into the body's rhythms, which are often much clearer than the perceptions of the mind. After all, we can't change what we don't know. While grieving, our awareness is often misguidedly placed on the drama of our losses. Increasing awareness of the body improves the receptivity of the mind because of the intricate union of these two aspects of our system.

Learning how our body responds to our actions is expertly demonstrated in the alternation of first feeling a joint in stillness and then feeling it in action. When we focus on how it feels to move this part of our body, we engage in feeling the effects more precisely.

The monitoring of the condition of our joints serves as a mapping device. It is a fresh angle on self-reflection, which enables us to witness progress. The moving body releases information regarding feelings and mental impressions that we hold in our molecules. By carefully listening to the emergence, we can hear our own internal guidance taking us a step closer to reinforcing existing feelings or changing them to suit our needs.

The flexions and extensions, contractions and torsions—all help the body purge undesired chemical byproducts of grief. These actions promote the release of toxins that, if left inside, make our anxiety greater, our depression deeper, and our confusion more pronounced. Monitoring the daily changes helps us witness the small improvements that practice of this technique brings. By witnessing these daily micro improvements, you can gain renewed hope in the possibility of incremental shifts that reduce classical negative anticipatory thinking.

The mind can conveniently "forget" some joints, so try to remember to not skip any of the exercises so as to avoid further blockages. Even if you can't move a joint due to a functional limitation, simply visualize the rotation. Once we've cleared the pathways of the life force in the system, we are ready to further stir up our feelings and make a deeper and more significant connection with them—something the following exercise, the Windmill, is uniquely suited for.

Whisking Up the Feelings

The Windmill is the key *asana* in the Yoga for Grief Relief *sadhana* and gives you access to the most powerful resource you can tap into. Although it is not found in classical yoga texts, it relates to a similar exercise included in Bioenergetics, a technique invented by American physician and psychotherapist Alexander Lowen (1994). I felt inspired to design the Windmill exercise and integrate it into my grief therapy practice because of the profound effect it had on me. As a somatic psychotherapist, I was absolutely fascinated by the immediate effect of how quickly whirling arm movements enhance the perception of feelings. In addition, I learned that in traditional Chinese medicine, some rotational movements of the arms are often prescribed to deal with symptoms of grief pinpointed in the lungs.

Ananda Balayogi Bhavanani, a dear friend and one of the modern scholars of Yoga in India, provided me with a Sanskrit name for the technique: *vayu chakram asana*, or "wheel of air." Through many years of using this technique, I have come to realize that the effectiveness of the Windmill is absolutely due to the intentionally direct contact with *anahata* chakra, the heart center, where attachment is developed.

Windmill (*Vayu Chakram Asana*)

Right Arm

1. Stand with your feet parallel, the knees unlocked, the spine straight, and your arms at your sides.

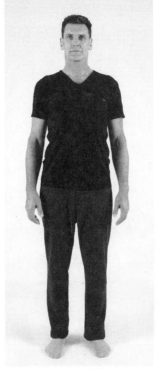
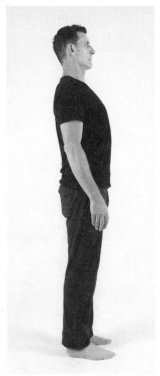

2. Turn the thumb of your right hand inward toward the leg first; then turn it backward, so that your pinky faces forward and your palm faces out to the side.

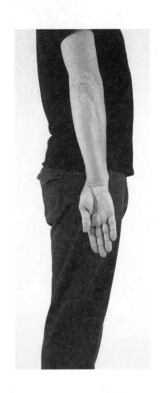

3. Inhale as you move your arm forward and up. Stop after the arm passes slightly behind the head and hold your breath, feeling the slight stretch in the pectoral muscles.

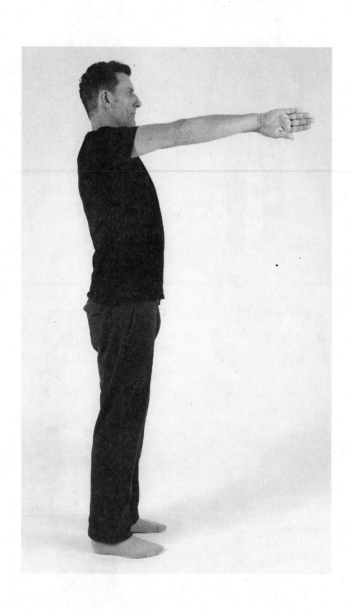

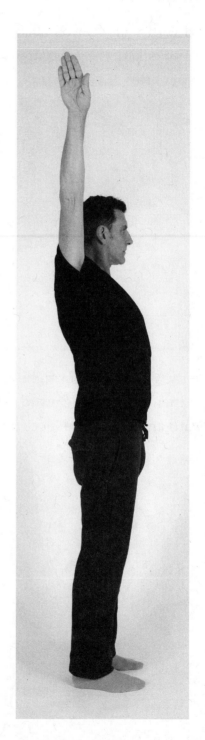

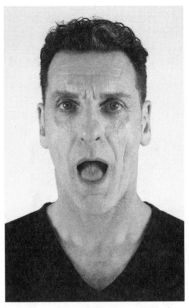

4. Open your mouth, relax your tongue, and, while exhaling, let the arm drop back and down while emitting an "aaah" sound. Avoid bumping your leg with your arm as it drops down in a free fall. Allow the arm to naturally stop swinging.

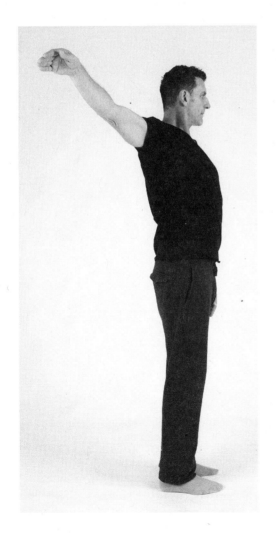

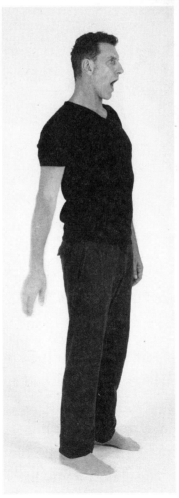

Semifast Form

1. After a number of repetitions of the slow form, bend your knees slightly and rotate your arm continuously at medium speed, following the same motion as before.

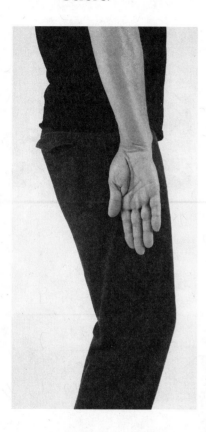

2. Allow for a quick inhalation through the nose followed by the "aaah" sound as you continuously rotate your arm. Make sure your arm rotates continuously. Avoid holding your breath as you did before. Avoid bobbing up and down; keep your knees bent throughout.

Fast Form

1. Increase the speed until you rotate the arm as fast as you can while continuing to breathe—more rapidly now—and making the "aaah" sound.

2. Stop the movement, straighten the knees, and connect with any emotions or feelings that might arise with closed eyes.

You might experience pain in your fingertips. If the pain is too intense, you may hold your arm upright and allow the blood to flow away from the extremities, which releases any pain almost immediately. Please also consider bearing with the pain, because it might be an effective metaphor for your willingness to withstand the pain of grief.

Left Arm

1. Repeat as for the right arm.

Both Arms

1. Face both palms out with the pinkies facing forward.

2. Inhale as you move both arms forward and up.

3. Stop the movement when the arms pass slightly behind your head. Hold your breath, feeling the slight stretch in both pectoral muscles.

4. Open your mouth, relax your tongue, and, while exhaling, let the arms drop back and down while emitting an "aaah" sound.

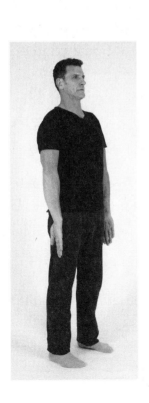
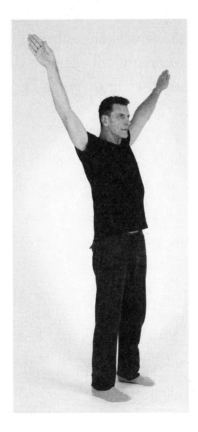
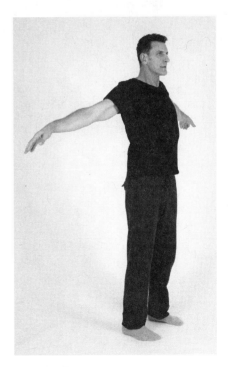

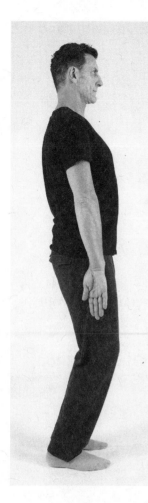

Semifast Form

1. After a number of repetitions of the slow form, bend your knees slightly and rotate both arms continuously at medium speed, following the same motion as before.

Fast Form

1. Increase the speed until you rotate the arms as fast as you can while continuing with the fast breath and the "aaah" sound.

2. Stop the movement, straighten the knees, and connect with any emotions or feelings that might arise with closed eyes.

Suggested number of repetitions: 10 times when performing the slow version; no less than 10 times when performing the semifast and fast versions. A better recommendation, however, is for you to simply self-regulate the repetitions, since counting them can distract from the upsurge of emotional content.

Benefits

- It unblocks the heart chakra, oxygenating and relaxing the pectoral muscles while allowing the feelings and emotions to find a way to the surface of your body and your consciousness.

- It enhances the upper-pectoral breath, increasing the lungs' capacity to receive air.

- It increases blood circulation to the upper thorax.

- It helps release tightness in the neck and lessen the sensation of feeling choked.

- It increases a general feeling of aliveness.

- It increases the sensation in the soles of your feet, allowing a deeper feeling of grounding.

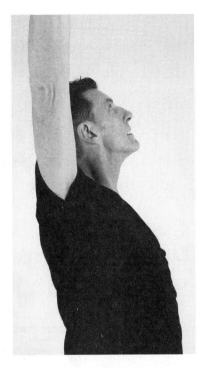

Precautions

- Ensure that the neck remains relaxed and the head stays straight throughout the exercise. Avoid tilting the head in any direction.

- Keep your knees bent (when practicing the semifast and fast forms) to reduce lower-back impact.

- Bear in mind that all degrees of practice—from visualization to full performance—are effective.

- Remember not to break the straight line of your posture as you exhale and bring the arms down.

- Do not twist the body to the side or rotate it while dropping the arms down as you exhale.

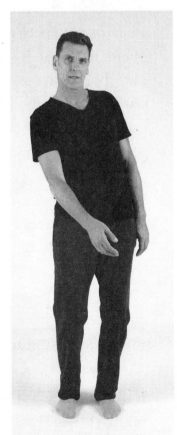

Contraindications

- Those suffering from rotator cuff–related conditions should only visualize the Windmill or perform it in a way that does not promote pain. If pain appears, stop movement, then try a simpler, less involved variation.

- The semifast and fast movements should be performed with care, respecting the inherent limitations with regard to any preexisting conditions such as neck, shoulder, or back injuries, or a heart condition. If any of these movements promote more than slight pain, or if you have doubts about whether they are appropriate for you at this time, please consult a medical professional before performing this exercise.

The Windmill helps activate the pectoral muscles while helping the scapulae to rotate, unlocking our emotional armor and relieving tension in the shoulder area. As the tense muscles start to loosen, our perceptions change as buried emotions start migrating from stuck places in the body.

The nature of the Windmill exercise is active. I feel it is important to emphasize that although it is natural to resist the emotions these movements might bring up, working through them is the only way to transform grief.

Practicing the Windmill proves helpful for what was once tense, locked, and shut away to become open and dynamic. You are invited to meet yourself fully when you activate this part of your body, enhancing the potential to alter your perception of your previously held beliefs.

Just like kids think they are invisible when they hide behind their own hands while playing peek-a-boo, we play an adult version of the game by thinking that by not naming our feelings and ignoring them, we don't feel them. We know that everybody can see the little kid behind his hands and, in a similar way, our higher self can see what we don't want to acknowledge as part of our experience. How can we change something when we don't know it is there? How can we consciously transform a belief if we are not aware of it?

Moving through the pain of grief is an essential task. Feeling the pain and becoming familiar with it is the first step. Next, we consciously work with the pain and transform it through our actions. Remember that you have not actually created any feelings by practicing the Windmill: they are already there inside of you.

The short moment of retention of the in-breath allows for an opportunity to match the body's present environment of overcharged feelings and tension that you are going through in life, and it prepares the system for the subsequent relief when swinging the arm back and down. The "aaah" sound induces your ability to express yourself, to get things off your chest. Sound helps open the pathways toward a full expression of the emotions associated with the loss and with the new situation that results. Because grieving individuals need to be heard, opening the avenues of communication both with yourself and others is very important. The Universe behaves as waves; using sound can help you begin to modify your reality on a cosmic level. Your ability to speak your truth reshapes the circumstances that compose your new reality.

During times of grief, acknowledging where we are in relation to our process can be challenging. Probably infused by the societal awkwardness around grief—the fact that nobody wants to talk about it—we too feel awkward and not necessarily comfortable exposing our aching hearts, showing our true pain. This promotes isolation and enhances the feeling that no one can understand us. While it is true that no two individuals grieve in the same way, it is also true that there are universal traits to everyone's grief, and sharing in this process can be of immense assistance at this time. Being able to speak about your reality when grieving can help you emotionally accept the reality of the loss. This is liberating in itself, provided that the other is a good listener. What is a good listener? Someone who is receptive, accepting, and willing to just listen and not give advice; someone who is not apt to give flippant answers such as, "Don't worry, you'll be all right!"

Some prefer the slow form of the Windmill because it is more pleasant than the semifast and fast forms. Preferably, the faster forms of the technique should be practiced with supervision and closely monitored by an experienced and seasoned yoga therapist or, even better, by a competent body-oriented psychotherapist. The elevated energetic tone of both the semifast and fast forms often evoke very intense feelings. The willingness and readiness to expose your deepest defense mechanisms demands increased caution, compassion, and care toward yourself.

I have seen many yoga practitioners having breakthroughs with the Windmill, tapping into their own unmasked hearts; at times exhilarated by merely witnessing their own rich palette of feelings, other times overwhelmed by the intensity of it all. Because the consequences can be very intense, I suggest using the slow form only at first. You may want to leave the other two speeds for a time when you can practice with proper guidance and are emotionally prepared to work with what arises. While it is true that you want to face your emotional reality, you must do so in a way that is feasible and productive for growth.

The image of a windmill using the power of the wind to grind grains into flour is as a valid analogy, as it exemplifies the process of working through our own grief. Transforming the hardness of the process into something we can derive nurturance from mirrors the hard shell on the grain. The milling turns the hardness into something that we can use. By releasing our armored posture of protection, we gain access to the hidden gem written about earlier in this chapter. Chapter 6 further addresses the aspects of such a transformation.

Let Go!

The Attitude of Discharging exercise offers an extraordinary outlet for your heightened feelings, brought to consciousness after practicing the Windmill. Now stirred up, your emotions are available and accessible for creative externalization.

This *asana* demonstrates how yoga can be used to address issues at their core by helping individuals discharge unwanted feelings. Instead of offering specific antidotes for each feeling, we efficiently assume an attitude of *letting go* to be applied to any and all feelings.

The question grieving individuals ask most often is, "What do I do with these feelings?" Even though feelings are to be felt, it is true that most of us want to do something with them. In the words of J. William Worden, "Sadness must be accompanied by an awareness of what one has lost, anger needs to be properly and effectively targeted, guilt needs to be evaluated and resolved, and anxiety needs to be identified and managed" (2009, 96).

Once you identify your feelings, you can assess what actions are needed to address them. The following *asana* allows you to discharge negative and unpleasant feelings, or perhaps to discharge those that prevent you from accessing the positive feelings you awaken by practicing the Windmill and would like to experience more deeply.

Attitude of Discharging (*Utthita Lolasana*)

1. Stand with legs apart, feet parallel, and knees bent.

2. On an inhale, bring the arms forward and up, then bend backward, moving the pelvis forward and tilting the head back.

3. Hold your breath at the end of the inhalation.

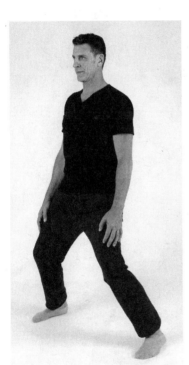 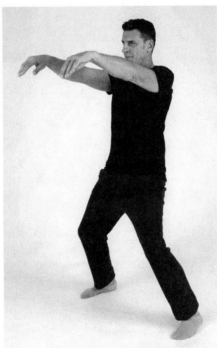 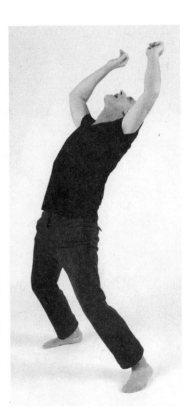

4. Open your mouth, relax the tongue, and then, while exhaling, swing the upper body forward and down until coming to a complete relaxation of the upper body and emitting an "aaah" sound.

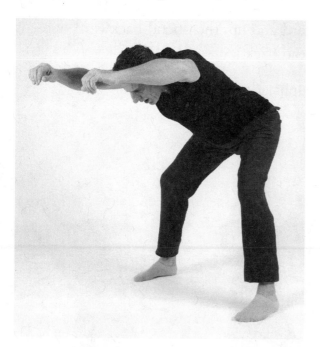
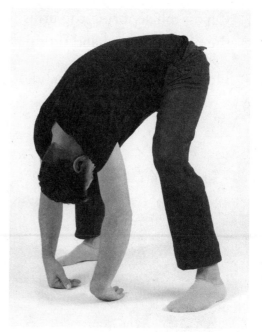

5. While inhaling, move the arms forward and up. Repeat.

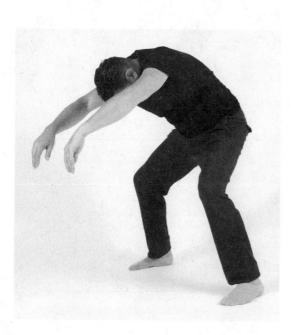
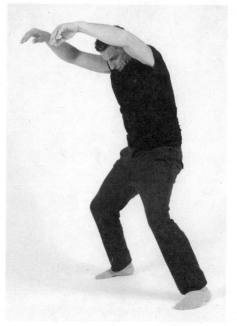

Suggested number of repetitions: 10 times.

Benefits

- It tones the spinal nerves.

- It massages the vital organs.

- It stretches the hamstrings and back muscles.

- It improves lymphatic movement and drainage from the abdomen and base of the lungs, allowing for an improved, fuller breath.

- It stimulates blood flow to the brain.

- It facilitates discharge, offering feelings and emotional sensations a way out.

Precautions

- Keep the knees bent at all times, including at the end of the inhalation when you are bent backward.

- Make sure the head and arms come to a full relaxation after each downward swinging movement when performing the regular version.

Contraindications

- This *asana* should be modified if practiced by people suffering from vertigo. In this case, avoid placing the head down.

- People with high blood pressure should avoid the complete version of the *asana*, limiting the forward-down movement with the upper torso.

- Those suffering from back conditions, particularly in the lower back, need to monitor pain especially when coming up after the downward swinging movement.

The difficult moment of bending backward at the end of the inhalation might mirror an equally challenging moment during bereavement: that of feeling exposed, awkward, imbalanced, vulnerable. The forceful downward movement offers an opportunity to release those embodied feelings.

I've found three variations of this posture to be particularly helpful to those who are grieving:

The first variation includes performing the technique in a continuous fashion and with no retention of the in-breath at the end of each inhalation. Always keep your knees bent to avoid locking them in an attempt to control the heightened intensity of feelings. In my practice, I've found that active people, and men in particular, usually enjoy this variation because of its enhanced active component. The constant use of the "aaah" sound also tends to resonate with men who usually prefer growling out their emotions to talking about them.

Suggested number of repetitions: 10 times.

A second variation entails "placing" the particular feeling you need to discharge in the palms of your hands. As you move forward and down, visualize that emotion being released into the earth. Holding the feeling in the palms helps the mind concretize the feeling and enhances the intensity and focus of the discharge.

Suggested number of repetitions: 10 times.

A third variation has your hands making full contact with the floor at the end of the exhalation, with the "aaah" sound sustained. Avoid tapping the hands on the floor; rather, keep the full contact for as long as you are exhaling and emitting the "aaah" sound. Visualize pushing the feelings forcefully into the hot magma at the center of the earth. Allow the upper body to fully lean on the hands and intensify the push, imagining the emotion traveling at high speed and melting into the earth's core. Remember that melting something does not get rid of it, it merely changes its form. In a similar way our feelings cannot disappear but instead can be transformed with intention, time, and work.

Suggested number of repetitions: 3 times.

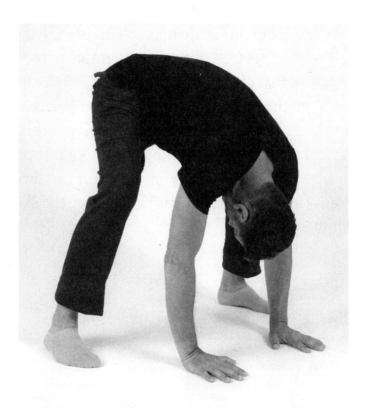

If you are compromised in your bodily capacity to perform this exercise, be safe and only engage up to your limit, or practice by visualizing the technique. I've even proposed this exercise to people confined to a wheelchair, engaging only the upper body, arms, and head as a variation of this posture.

After performing such an intense *asana*, we are now ready to move to a quieter, calmer practice to continue working with our grief.

Sleep Better and Awaken to a New Perspective

The technique that follows is useful to help balance the pineal gland. Because of its involvement in regulating the functions of the other endocrine glands, this is a good way to reset the endocrine system in its entirety. This exercise can help individuals strengthen their protection from foreign agents and avoid the relapse of preexisting conditions that often occurs at this vulnerable time. This is due to the relationship between the endocrine system and the immune system, particularly at the thymus gland. The pineal gland is often heavily taxed during the grief process, and the insomnia many grievers experience—or its opposite, oversleeping—is the result of an imbalance in the melatonin it produces. Engaging the optic nerves is a way of addressing this disturbance, since the gland reacts to light registered through these nerves.

Concentrated Gazing (*Tratak*)

1. Sit comfortably and extend your right arm with your fist closed and your thumb pointing up, the thumbnail facing you. If you need support for the arm, place the closed fist of your left hand at the right armpit. You may also bend the right knee and use your knee to support the arm.

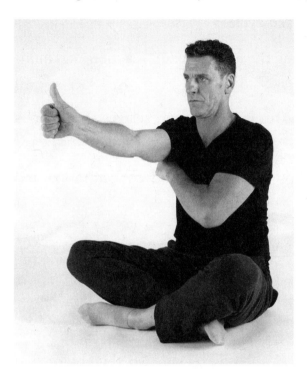 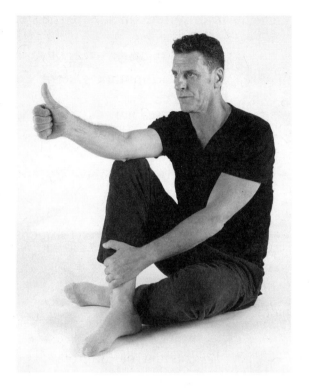

2. Locate a distant object (at least 10 feet away) at eye level as a focal point, and place your thumbnail within the line of vision between your eyes and the distant object of focus. The object being focused on should be relatively small, such as a doorknob, a rock, or a drawn black dot.

3. Focus on your thumbnail for 1 minute.

4. Shift your focus to the distant object for 1 minute.

5. Shift back to your thumbnail.

6. Repeat the process of switching the focus 3 times (6 times in total). Avoid blinking throughout the exercise if you can.

Suggested time: Including 1 minute of focus and three switches between focal points, the practice takes 6 minutes.

Benefits

- It stimulates the optic nerves, which prompts the functions of the pineal gland. The resulting balanced levels of melatonin tend to regulate many biorhythms, including the sleep-wake cycle.

- It helps regulate stress by influencing the fight-or-flight reaction, and modulates the immune system.

- It increases nervous stability, removes insomnia, and relaxes the anxious mind.

- It improves the memory and helps to develop good concentration and strong willpower.

- Spiritually, it awakens *ajna* chakra.

Precautions

- Always avoid unnecessary strain.

- Be tolerant of different experiences such as seeing two thumbs or two distant focal points—these experiences change with time.

Contraindications

- Those suffering from glaucoma should be sensitive to pain and modify the practice as needed, by reducing the time focusing or the number of changes between focal points.

Many practitioners report falling asleep before completing a full round of Concentrated Gazing. With steady practice, cosmic rhythms soothe the body, helping it remember when to sleep and when to stay awake. The wisdom of healthy grieving lives more in the Spirit than in the mind. Working with the pineal gland is important for its connection with *ajna* chakra, the third eye, where we view life through awakened intuitive knowledge. Our Spirit knows that things end, and our bodies are accustomed to processing endings constantly, yet it is our minds that want the things we are attached to to be with us forever.

Concentrated Gazing also offers a symbolic opportunity to take a look at how we want to transition through the next steps of our lives. The two focal points, one close and one distant, serve as symbols of the situations we go through when grieving. When the old reality is not there any longer and the new one is not yet known, our controlling minds have a hard time waiting. The negative anticipatory thinking indicative of the limbic system's involvement in grief makes us perceive the projected new reality negatively. It fills us with ideas such as thinking that no one will love us as much or that no job will ever suit us in the same way. That might be true, or completely false, and we can't know yet. In the meantime, we can only trust the journey and accept that change will come. Shifting focus from the thumbnail (our present situation) to the chosen distant point (the new reality to be discovered) symbolizes the journey ahead.

Deciding on what could be the distant focal point can be very useful in determining the next steps of the journey. You can choose a picture representative of how you would like to feel in the future, or the house you would like to have, or the job you would like to get. Place it in the distance, so when you switch to that focal point, you are adding intention and meaning to your practice. Deciding where to start and where to end (with the distant or close focal point) can add strength to your ability to meet yourself where you are and to your precision in defining your future.

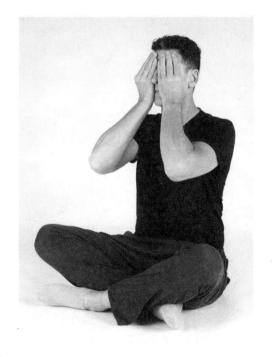

Sometimes the eyes get tired or strained when practicing this technique. If this happens, rub the palms of your hands together, then bring the cupped hands to your eyes and enjoy the warmth and darkness that can soothe them.

After acknowledging the reality of your loss, identifying where you are in the present moment, and beginning to understand where you would like to be in the future, you can practice a technique that helps you control your immediate environment and effectively calms the mind.

Control Is Somehow Possible

One of the realities of grief is that, in most cases, the loss was probably out of our control. Even when the loss is the result of a choice, the subsequent suffering is often unavoidable. If we had complete control we would never lose anything, nor would we choose to suffer.

When confronting the challenges of grief, the mind and the body both go through symptoms that mimic our discomfort when faced with loss of control (difficulty breathing, muscle tension, etc.). By actively engaging both mind and body through yoga exercises, we can immediately bring back some sense of control into our lives. Our most immediate connection to life is our breath, and bringing balance to it can be achieved by practicing Alternate-Nostril Breathing.

Alternate-Nostril Breathing (*Nadi Shodhana Pranayama*)

You may not know it, but the right nostril and the left nostril rarely carry the same amount of air. Try this simple exercise: lick your index finger, inhale, and bring your finger close to your right nostril while exhaling, then repeat with the other nostril. Well? Unless you are in deep balance at this time, one of them carries more air than the other.

1. Sit in a comfortable position with the head and spine upright and the left arm bent over your belly so that the right elbow can rest on the left forearm.

2. Hold the fingers of your right hand in front of your face. Rest the index and middle fingers gently on the center of the eyebrows. Both fingers should be relaxed. Position the thumb next to the right nostril and the ring finger next to the left nostril. The little finger should be comfortably folded.

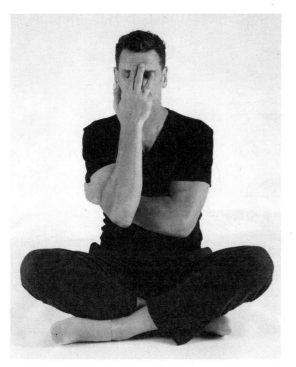 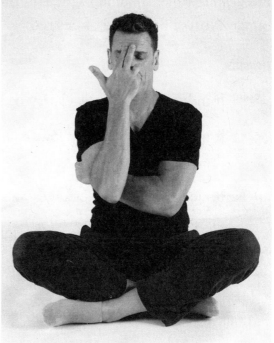

3. Inhale, then close the left nostril with the ring finger and exhale through the right nostril.

4. Inhale through the same right nostril.

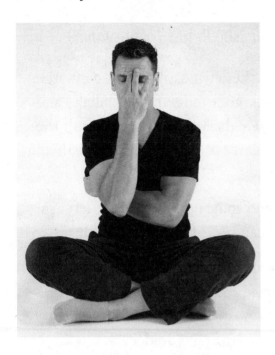

5. Unblock the left nostril and close the right one with the thumb.

6. Exhale through the left nostril.

7. Inhale through the same nostril, the left.

8. Unblock the right nostril and close the left one with your ring finger.

9. Exhale through the right nostril and inhale through the same nostril.

10. Continue the alternation, only changing nostrils after the inhalation.

Suggested time: 5 minutes of Alternate-Nostril Breathing, plus 5 minutes of Single-Nostril Breathing, if desired.

Benefits

- It induces tranquility, clarity of thought, and concentration.

- It increases vitality and lowers levels of stress and anxiety by balancing the flow of life force.

- It clears life force blockages and balances the flow in both nostrils.

- Carbon dioxide is efficiently expelled and the blood is purified of toxins.

- It promotes spiritual awakening.

Precautions

- Avoid forcing the breath.

- Do not breathe through the mouth.

- Sometimes one nostril may be blocked, preventing the easy flow of breath. If the right nostril is blocked, make a fist with your left hand and place it under your right armpit. Press up against the underarm, bringing your right arm down. Continue to practice this way for 3 minutes. Then, remove the hand. Repeat for the left side, as necessary.

Contraindications

- None.

In yoga, the right nostril relates to the sun: masculinity, activity, giving, daytime, extroversion, social life, partying. The left relates to the moon: femininity, passivity, receiving, nighttime, introversion, spiritual life, resting. When experiencing anxiety, your right nostril is more engaged; the opposite occurs when you are depressed or depleted—the left nostril carries more air. Making the air go through both nostrils alternately brings your system into a more balanced relationship between your active and passive aspects of the self, influencing the way you experience the present situation. It allows the mind to calm and tap into the alternation of all things. This can help you trust that even though you are now anxious, you will eventually relax; and if you are sad, you will eventually be happy again.

The right nostril also corresponds to the sympathetic, energizing branch of the autonomic nervous system. The left nostril is related to the relaxing parasympathetic branch that usually prevails when one is grieving. Balancing the activity of these two aspects of your nervous system reestablishes the lost equilibrium, regulating your functions and balancing your reactions. This is assuredly a much more stable way to respond to your new environment.

Practicing breathing through a single nostril—provided that it's not done for more than 5 minutes—can bring surprising changes to your emotional state, energizing you when you're feeling depressed and calming you when you're feeling anxious. Mentally, you can gain a more positive perspective or calm the constant chatter of thoughts with Alternate-Nostril Breathing. Given the power of this technique, the directive of doing a maximum of 5 minutes' work with one nostril is to be taken seriously. Please know that exceeding 5 minutes' time can result in difficulties negotiating the altered state and rebalancing your energy properly.

In general, retaining the breath, either in or out, is another possible manipulation of the breath when practicing *pranayama*. On a psychological level it helps us perceive and deal with two opposite types of anxieties: retaining the in-breath relates to the anxiety we experience related to life, to its fullness, to its intensity; retaining the out-breath relates to our feelings about death in general, and particularly our own deaths. While practicing Alternate-Nostril Breathing, notice if you are holding your breath at the end of the inhalation or the exhalation, and see if it relates to your feelings.

Voluntarily manipulating the active and passive within you helps you accept that change is the norm, that all things fluctuate, and that change is possible within yourself. No matter where you are in your grieving process, you will not be in the same place in the future, regardless of what things look like in the present moment. Switching willingly from one nostril to the other and witnessing the change helps your mind integrate the new situation as part of your ever-changing life.

After witnessing the varying symptoms of grief and starting to use your breath to bring back a sense of control, you are now ready to fully relax.

Bringing Calm to a Scattered Mind and a Distressed Body

Grief is stressful. Therefore, a state of relaxation is crucial; and yet this state is difficult to access most of the time. The stress-relieving effects of yoga are some of the most studied features of the discipline and are very useful when grieving. Even though any relaxation technique could work and would be good, my intention in including a self-relaxation technique is to empower individuals to use their own means to relax. The first lesson of loss is to not depend on the permanence of things—which is why an external source of relaxation, such as soothing music or a guided relaxation on a DVD, while beneficial, would not use the newly acquired information to our maximum benefit.

Self-Relaxation Technique (*Anga Shaithilya*)

1. Lie on your back, with your palms facing up. Bring your awareness to the breath. Find the natural rhythm of your breath, breathing in and out slowly and steadily through the nostrils.

2. Now bring the awareness to your feet.

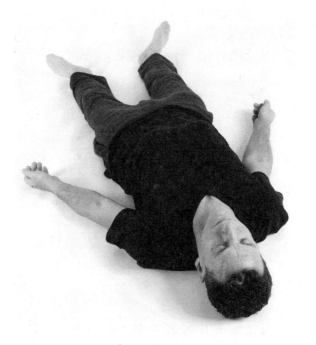

3. Inhale, exhale.

4. Inhale, exhale, repeating to yourself silently, "My feet are relaxed."

5. Bring awareness to your legs.

6. Inhale, exhale. While exhaling, repeat silently to yourself, "My legs are relaxed."

7. Bring awareness to your pelvis.

8. Inhale, exhale. While exhaling, repeat silently to yourself, "My pelvis is relaxed."

9. Continue the practice by repeating the same pattern for:

   - Hands

   - Arms

   - Shoulders

   - Back

   - Torso

   - Neck

- Face

- Head

- Mind

10. End by repeating internally, "I am completely relaxed" three times.

Suggested time: 10 minutes.

Benefits

- It relaxes the body.

- It helps the mind relax.

- It combats the stressful effects of grief.

- It replenishes the general energy level of the body, combating fatigue.

Precautions

- Do your best to memorize the twelve body parts included in the technique to avoid distractions while practicing it.

Contraindications

- None.

Using a technique that offers relaxation with deep detailed awareness of oneself and that is grounded in the rhythm of the breath is a great way to integrate other exercises of the practice in the relaxation. Notice that this exercise follows the same body order as the Energy Flow Series. Opening the practice with the directive to stay connected with your breath rhythm is another form of Breath Meditation. The repetition of "My _____ is/are relaxed" is nothing other than the active practice of Resolve (see the following exercise).

Be prepared to hear the mind voicing statements such as "I can't relax because I have to remember what part is next." To remedy this, memorize the parts before practicing and you can avoid this interruption. This technique helps with many of the symptoms of grief including physical pain. It gives the body an opportunity to take a rest from the depleting hyperactive symptoms of the emotional stress and replenish itself. Relaxing the body also helps the mind calm down and reduce the constant mental chatter, allowing you to focus on planting the seeds of your new life through Resolve.

Dissolving Old Patterns and Reprogramming the Mind with Intention

Yoga acknowledges the principle of *pronoia*, a neologism coined by modern philosophers expressing an old truth. It states that the Universe is conspiring in our highest good. This is the polar opposite of *paranoia*, which, in essence, involves the belief that the Universe is conspiring against us.

For most of humanity, the latter concept prevails as an accurate description of a world that is not at all supportive and comes after us loaded with jeopardizing intentions. Yoga recognizes this as false and makes it clear that the whole process starts with an idea in our mind. Yoga states, "We create the mold and then the Universe is in charge of filling it up."

Resolve (*Sankalpa*)

The translation of the word *sankalpa* is "resolve" or "resolution." It refers to the application of willpower through a conscious decision-making process. It takes the form of a short mental statement, which is imprinted by repetition on the subconscious mind. *Sankalpa* influences the way things are to happen with determination and intention.

The statement represents a mold that, once created, allows for the providential powers of the Universe to help manifestation occur. Remember, you are the only one actually capable of making your own mold. The word *sankalpa* refers to both the name of the technique as well as the content of the statement itself.

1. Think of the perfect way in which you want an intention to manifest and then state it in a succinct phrase that:

   - is expressed in present tense.

   - avoids using the word "no" or terms that express negative concepts. For example, "I will not be single" should be replaced with "I am married."

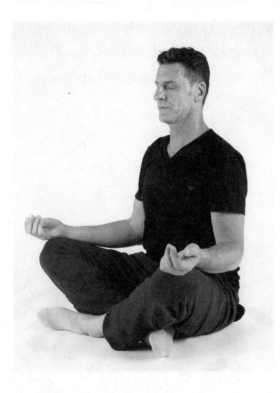

2. Sit comfortably with your hands on your knees. Breathe normally, acknowledging any outside thought that arises and let it go. Inhale, then on the exhale say your statement to yourself, being fully present with each individual word of the statement. (You may pause after each word.)

3. Take a deep breath and move to the next repetition. With your eyes closed, continue repeating your statement. Then breathe in and out once without repeating the statement. When done, open your eyes.

Suggested number of repetitions: 3 times.

The concept this technique refers to is in the core of the old saying "Ask and ye shall be given," to which I'd like to add, "if it is in the order of things." Why?

Many people ask for things that are not within the Universal order and then blame the system, rather than acknowledging that their ignorance of the order is the real reason things did not manifest. By "the order," I mean the systematic and precise way in which things work in the Universe and that is reflected in such truths as "Nothing is permanent." All things end, regardless of whether we are thinking of a vase, a day, or a thought. Without this acknowledgment, when asking for something to remain, the mechanism sparked by *sankalpa* will not work and the Universe will not support our petition. If I'm fifty-four, I can ask for "youthful fifties," but I can't ask to be fifteen again—it simply won't happen!

By clearly identifying what to ask for, and how to phrase it, we engage in a simple way of jump-starting the process of manifestation. Even though most of us have wants, it is surprisingly hard for people to actually express their wishes in an exact way! In my years of using Resolve, I have had to work diligently to help individuals identify what they want by spending hours sorting through all kinds of misunderstandings, old programming, and stale beliefs.

Prior to identifying what we want, we usually name what we don't want, what we fear, why we should not want it, and so forth. This means that our minds are absolutely full of all these other considerations, and, in the meantime, the Universe is busy filling up the corresponding molds as it competently does.

This is why we manifest what we fear and this is also how we manifest what we don't want. As you might know, "You can never get enough of what you really don't want!" If your mental programming—and created mold—is "I'm not going to get that job" or "I'd love to get that job, but there are so many others who are better prepared," then the Universe will accommodate you with an opportunity of losing that job. It might seem like an extremely minuscule semantic deviation, but the consequences resulting from such misunderstandings are also extremely clear. (See the sidebar that follows, "Aiding the Practice Through Journaling," for an effective approach to naming what we want.)

To say "I am not unhappy" is very different from saying "I am happy," and believe me, the Universe is listening precisely. To understand why precision is important, let me share with you an old story from India.

Aiding the Practice Through Journaling

As a simple exercise, think about what you want, and write your statement describing it; then continue to write down each modification of the statement as you develop it. Make no judgments, write no "shoulds"—just write what comes up. You will probably see a pathway, a mental road map that you have been following, that will reveal your misconceptions. Keep in mind that when you arrive at the "right" statement, a subtle "eye-smile" appears, a slight widening of your forehead accompanied by a sense of "Eureka! This is it!" That feeling is clearly identifiable, no questions asked, no doubts about it—it is resonating inside of you as accurate. Until that aha moment of recognition, keep working on your authentic expression, your personal Resolve. Know that you are actually working on your innermost wishes and that you are ultimately determining your future!

After you have come up with your statement and you are practicing repeating it, I suggest you also journal the internal responses and considerations your mind comes up with. It is normal to listen to the internal voice challenging your statements with phrases that denote the adverse reality, the one you are trying to modify. Since the manifestation process is happening regardless, if the statement is "I have a partner" and the mind comes up with "You are lying, no one would love you!" the idea/mold ready to be filled up is the latter. You may discover that what's written actually reveals your present mental programming: that you are really not worth loving.

By attending to your body, calming your mind, and exploring the nature of your desires on a deeper level, you are now truly ready to go within, to practice Breath Meditation and leave everything up to the Universe.

A couple, both age sixty and still married after forty years, find a genie lamp. When they rub it, the genie appears and comes to life. The genie speaks, "Lady, your wishes shall be granted. What would you like?"

"I want enough money to go around the world twice with my husband," the woman responds. In an instant, the genie manifests a briefcase full of enough money for the both of them to go around the world twice.

The genie then turns to the gentleman and says, "Sir, your wishes too shall be granted. What would you like?"

"I'd like to have a wife thirty years younger than me!" replies the opportunist. The genie then responds by turning the man into a ninety-year-old!

The lesson of this story is to be very clear and precise when asking for what you want; otherwise you may end up getting what you really don't want. Resolve is the mechanism that kick-starts the process of manifestation. Thoughtfully identifying and defining an idea can and will act as a guiding principle, a light-house in the darkness of your emotional storm. Then your actions, thoughts, and speech can aim in the proper direction and start bringing to fruition what until now has lived only within the realm of your wishes.

Opening to Spirit

This meditation technique can be seen as the simplest of all breathing exercises, the basis of all our work. Besides the spiritual benefits and effects, staying with your own breath is a powerful way of being present and in deep connection with your life, not drawn in by the past or contemplating the future.

Breath Meditation

1. Sit in a comfortable position, with the spine straight and the hands resting on your knees with the palms facing upward.

2. Stay still.

3. Bring awareness to your breath. Feel the air going in and out softly through your nostrils.

4. Remain present for each inhalation and each exhalation.

5. As the mind drifts off, bring it back to your breath. As if you are placing paper boats on a stream of water, place the distracting thoughts in the outgoing stream of the exhalation.

6. Remain concentrated on your breath, and only on your breath, exhaling each distracting thought.

Suggested time: 5 to 10 minutes.

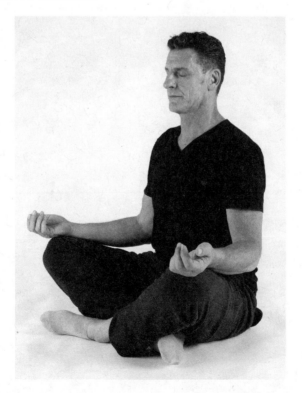

Although it is an extremely simple technique, the execution can prove to be quite difficult. Your ability to remain concentrated on the breath is permanently challenged by your very active body and unstoppable mind. You can start full of intention and find yourself out on a limb after only a few breath cycles.

Fortunately, your breath is constant and your need to take the next in-breath is unavoidable, so bringing the mind back to the breath is relatively simple. Keep coming back to the breath; with time, you'll see that your departures are scarcer, and that as you stay with your breath a certain sense of calmness and fulfillment appears.

You are now developing the skill to stay present with yourself, to keep yourself company and bring ease when feeling abandoned. I've stated before that, when grieving, you should focus first on the Spirit, because the body is profoundly engaged in its reaction and the mind is shattered and scattered. For this reason, meditation and its ability to help you connect with your Spirit become a key element of the practice. Though meditation can be challenging when you are experiencing acute grief, it is an activity that will gently lead you to the source of knowledge you intend to tap into.

Now that you have read how to perform each practice and understand generally how the techniques serve to allay some of the symptoms of grief, you probably want to get started and figure out how to incorporate these practices into your life. There are some important questions to ponder as you start to integrate some of these exercises into a personal practice.

The next chapter considers what exercises you should include, how much time you should spend practicing, whether you should practice by yourself or seek help, how long you should practice, and other practical details. Whether you are an experienced yoga practitioner or just starting out, whether you have just begun to cope with some of your grief symptoms or at the end of the process, the next chapter will help you to integrate the techniques into your personal practice.

CHAPTER 5

Designing the Logistical Aspects of Your Practice

There is a famous quote usually attributed to the great German philosopher Johann Wolfgang von Goethe (1749–1832):

"Until one is committed, there is hesitancy, the chance to draw back. Concerning all acts of initiative (and creation), there is one elementary truth, the ignorance of which kills countless ideas and splendid plans: that the moment one definitely commits oneself, then Providence moves too. All sorts of things occur to help one that would never otherwise have occurred. A whole stream of events issues from the decision, raising in one's favor all manner of unforeseen incidents and meetings and material assistance, which no man could have dreamed would have come his way. **Whatever you can do, or dream you can do, begin it.** Boldness has genius, power, and magic in it" (emphasis added).

What a beautiful way of presenting the universal principle of pronoia! It explains the mechanism of manifestation and emphasizes a key aspect: to commit to what we want. The resulting actions actually help the brain reshape itself: this is neuroplasticity at its best! Through the fruits of our commitment we can establish new neuronal connections that will lead us not to where we think we should be or where we don't desire to be, but where we truly want to be.

As you now ponder how to implement the techniques I shared in the previous chapter and embark on your personal practice, I "re-mind" you that your commitment is essential. By accepting your limitations and needs, you are actually making your commitment feasible. Be realistic, commit to what you can, and do it!

Setting the Intention

There are two philosophical concepts found in *The Yoga Sutras of Patanjali* that can be translated as "practice." The first one, *abhyasa*, refers to a more general, all-encompassing method of practice that involves lifestyle choices, thoughts, speech, and actions. *Abhyasa* brings us greater tranquility or peace of mind. *Sadhana*, the second concept, can also be defined as practice, but it pertains to the actual techniques or exercises that are performed on a regular basis to achieve an overall enhancement of well-being. Taken together, these concepts can help us understand what it means to truly practice yoga.

As you begin to apply the traditional movements, breathing exercises, and cleansing techniques, setting aside an hour, a half hour, or whatever time you can dedicate to establishing a regular practice, you may realize that each breath can be an opportunity for transformation. My hope is that as you integrate these techniques into your daily life, your life itself becomes the practice.

Should You Practice Alone or Under Guidance?

Just as you are a solitary being in the midst of a crowded city street, practice is personal regardless of how many more are practicing with you. In ancient times, practicing yoga based on a book like the one you are reading, without live contact with a teacher, master, or guru, was unthinkable. Even though yoga was commonly passed down within the context of the family, from one generation to the next, there is an essential trinity thought to lead to a successful spiritual journey. It includes the individual (you), God or Spirit, and the guru—the one who leads the way after having walked it himself many times before.

In today's world people may practice through the guidance of a book or by following instructions provided on a DVD or a how-to video on the Internet. It is an essential principle in yoga therapy that the interaction with a therapist who can monitor the student's practice is an important aspect, adding strength to the techniques and ensuring safety for the Yoga practitioner.

Grief is so powerful that, in working with the dynamics activated by the Yoga techniques, it would be advisable to seek out a qualified professional at first. By "qualified," I mean either a yoga therapist well versed in grief counseling, or a grief counselor or therapist knowledgeable about yoga and its use in the therapeutic process. Because yoga has been embraced by a number of professionals in recent years, other therapists such as social workers, hospice nurses, chaplains, and others who work with grief-related issues can be trusted sources for guiding you through this work. Even a financial adviser who understands about the physical symptoms of grief and how to address them can mean the difference between wealth and poverty when, for example, dealing with finances after a divorce. Such a therapist—while encouraging a student to practice at home, encountering the "teacher within"—would also help him or her navigate the difficult emotions encountered in the grieving process.

Yoga practice can be a very subjective experience, often having different results in different settings. Should you decide to do the practice on your own, without professional guidance, remember to be sensitive and respectful of your needs and abilities. Monitor the effects of the techniques so you can use them appropriately when needed. Tune into the results, charting them as a valid indicator of the development of your process.

Is It Better to Practice Individually or in a Group?

While all yoga is therapeutic, yoga therapy thrives on personal individualized practice, especially at the beginning stages of the therapeutic process. Working with a qualified therapist familiar with integrating yoga as part of his or her toolbox is wholeheartedly advised. Either in a group setting, provided such a group is available in your community, or privately, choose whichever better suits your needs.

Working individually provides focused attention to treatment, offers input on adapting your practice to meet specific needs, and avoids interference from others in a class. On the other hand, practicing in a group allows you to witness other bereaved individuals grieve in ways that may be both profoundly different and strikingly similar to yours. Combating the tendency to isolate, this aspect of socialization can help normalize your relationship to your own grief while offering a support network.

In my Yoga for Grief Relief groups, all three aspects commonly found in traditional grief support groups are included: education, support, and social networking. Education serves the purpose of normalizing grief by sharing general information regarding the grieving process. We also look at how grief is addressed in different cultures and time periods. Support is established within the environment the group provides. It encourages authentic communication regarding our grief and serves to model healthy interactions to be replicated in the outside world. The social networking aspect encourages positive personal interactions that increase well-being for those of us listening as well as those sharing. When one is feeling depleted and without much to give, lending an ear to those expressing their grief can be an empowering experience.

Is It Safe to Do This Practice by Yourself?

Most of the techniques can be practiced safely on your own provided you read the sections dedicated to contraindications. Please identify any present condition that may require caution when you practice the exercises. This makes a tremendous difference between an exercise benefiting you or being harmful to you.

That said, the Windmill is the one exercise for which discretion must be used when practicing alone. The Windmill is a key technique of the program, and although the slow version is safe for most individuals, the semifast and fast versions of the Windmill quickly access deeply held emotions and buried physical feelings. I suggest that a competent professional trained in this work should monitor both the practice itself as well as the outcomes. If you are working with a yoga-savvy counselor, then your therapy provides an outlet for sharing your experience after practicing at home. The Windmill is the most active exercise, and the one best able to bring strong feelings to the surface. The emotions elicited during the grieving process are the raw materials you use for transformation.

Some of you might have an existing personal yoga practice and want to add some of my recommended techniques to your routine. Although this can certainly be effective, keep in mind that the truest benefits of this program occur when practiced sequentially in its entirety. By experiencing the routine fully, you can then effectively assess what to add to your practice and why. If you choose to embark on a solo practice, then you need to consider some of the following important logistical details.

Which Exercises Are Best for Me?

Whether to perform the entire practice or parts of it depends on what you would like to accomplish, how much time you have, and how much knowledge you possess of yoga and of yourself. The entire practice can be accomplished in ninety minutes and is inherently balanced, covering issues that most grieving individuals need.

Complete Breathing prepares your mind and body for the magnitude of the grieving process; the Energy Flow Series creates the conditions for healing and draws your awareness within; the Windmill brings feelings and sensations to the surface, sparking the process of transforming your grief into a source of self-knowledge; Attitude of Discharging offers an outlet for the raw available emotions; Concentrated Gazing promotes mental focus to restore the normal circadian rhythms; while Alternate-Nostril Breathing offers breath control to effectively bring balance and calm to your mind. The Self-Relaxation Technique helps decrease the stressful effects of grief, allowing optimal conditions for reprogramming your mind through Resolve, which uses the newly acquired knowledge to begin to construct a new identity. Finally you are ready to sit still in meditation to deepen the connection with your Spirit.

Practicing the entire sequence offers you the exponential effect of the combined benefits of the techniques. Yet, you may be better off practicing only certain parts as you begin to familiarize yourself with the work. Make sure you check with your physician before engaging in practice; keep in mind that yoga therapy is not a substitute for medical attention.

Becoming familiar with each technique and its effects on you gives you the confidence to choose which one works for what is troubling you. Again, I reiterate: your mind is best addressed through breath work, your body is helped most by physical postures, and your Spirit thrives with meditation. Yoga techniques influence all three aspects of your being. You can choose from each realm and come up with a combination that best suits your personal journey. Trust your instinct and inner wisdom to guide you.

Where Should I Practice?

While it is true that yoga is best practiced in a clean and calm environment, at least two hours after your last meal, wearing comfortable clothes, far from the chaos of the world, for at least ninety minutes, these perfect conditions are rarely met. The main criteria for understanding how to engage in the practice should always be "to meet yourself exactly where you are." You can then figure out which exercises to practice, where to situate yourself, when to practice, and how much time you can set aside to practice.

If you don't have a room dedicated for practice, then move some furniture around to create a suitable space, and bring in any objects or images that help you connect with your intention. This process exemplifies locating a new space inside of yourself. Sometimes when we feel "all over the place" in our mind, just cleaning and reorganizing our house starts to positively affect our emotional integration. Ordering our immediate surroundings often helps to calm down the internal disarray. Candles, incense, soothing music, and low light may provide you with supportive harmonizing associations to make your practice more meaningful.

Be flexible regarding where you practice, allowing for variations according to your life's circumstances. For example, if you are interviewing for a job that could ease pressing economic needs, then practice some calming breath work in the waiting room. If you find yourself struggling with road rage, pull over, stop the car, and practice Left-Nostril Breathing. Then get back on the road when you are calm and have lost sight of that annoying tailgater—you don't want to lose control and cause yourself more grief!

Sometimes it is good to enhance your practice by being outdoors connecting with nature and bringing in a sense of expansion. Conversely, if doing this seems too vulnerably open and distracting and lacks the intimacy you need, then practice where you can more easily accomplish the results you are after.

When Should I Practice?

Starting the day with an extended practice, deliciously dedicated to oneself, is not a luxury we all have. Feel free to do what you can in the morning, then add or repeat something in the middle of the day, and then practice before going to bed.

The Energy Flow Series is a great way to both start and end the day. In the morning it feels energizing, and at night calming, preparing you for a good night's sleep. The Windmill practice will elevate the general tone of your life force energy in the morning. The Attitude of Discharging exercise will help you discharge some of the extra tension accumulated during the day, if done in the late afternoon. Alternate-Nostril Breathing is a great midday practice that brings balance to your wildly fluctuating emotions. Concentrated Gazing works efficiently to put you to sleep at night and, if used in the morning, it resets the endocrine system, decreasing mood swings. (This may be especially important for women during bereavement to stabilize and reestablish balance in their endocrine system and counteract the common disturbances grief imposes on their normal menstrual cycle.) Choosing the right time to practice helps you adjust to your new environment more skillfully and helps to prepare you for the multitude of changes and new conditions in your life. From your first in-breath when you are born to your last out-breath at the moment of death, the time elapsed is all yours. The decisions you make regarding how to spend that time are also yours. Use your practice time wisely, so it reflects your sense of ownership of your time and your respect for it.

For How Long Should I Practice?

Finally, in terms of how long to practice each technique or how long your overall practice should be, let me just say this: something is better than nothing! Our systems react to all we do and all we think, so do what you can. It is true that for best results Alternate-Nostril Breathing should be practiced for no less than five minutes, yet a minute alone would also do some work. A minimum of three repetitions is better when practicing the Energy Flow Series, but one repetition also has benefits. What is optimal is to use whatever time you might have; just keep in mind that the more you practice, the deeper the effects will be.

An exception should be made with Single-Nostril Breathing. Practicing for more than five minutes can render stronger effects than you may desire. When practicing Left-Nostril Breathing, for example, you want to feel calmer, not depleted! It is okay to practice for more than five minutes if needed; just make sure you break it down with a minute or two of Alternate-Nostril Breathing.

The *sadhana* practice—in its entirety, and following the guidelines proposed for each technique in chapter 4—should take approximately ninety minutes. Please remember that, according to the variations and modifications you need to make, your practice time will vary. Supplementary techniques such as journaling and others offered in chapter 6 will also alter your personal practice time.

Becoming familiar with the techniques will allow you to know more easily what to call upon and when. With regular practice, the effects of the techniques will come alive in you and will even help you choose what to practice and when. Be sensitive to the daily fluctuations in your actual ability to engage in the techniques. If you spent a half hour doing *pawanmuktasana* yesterday and your muscles are sore today, reduce the time and intensity of the exercise to what you can tolerate.

Your Practice Changes as You Do

Please be open to the fact that you are undergoing constant change, and therefore your practice must shift as well to reflect your new needs and abilities. The grieving process and the tasks of mourning are not linear: your grief changes your practice and your practice changes your grief. There is wisdom in letting your practice reflect your state of being and adapting it accordingly. The way you practice is the way you live; what you practice now shapes your life. Be mindful of addressing your practice with the same grace and dignity that you want for yourself.

Perhaps it is accurate to say that you did not sign up for being where you are now, and yet, here you are. Practice jump-starts the process of transformation. See yourself functioning as the best operator of these tools by asking what you want to accomplish, listening to your voice, hearing your body's expression of its innate wisdom, and sensing what you need to do for yourself today—do something to commit to what you want.

CHAPTER 6

The Process of Transformation

Lyn Prashant, the founder of Integrative Grief Therapy, states that "we don't get over our losses, we change relationship to them." And she adds that "grief is our most available, untapped emotional resource for personal transformation" (2005). I wholeheartedly agree with her.

While honoring our personal losses, and mourning the relationship that once was, the transformation that we are talking about, in essence, is our own. As we begin to witness the appearance of our new self, we slowly recognize the cumulative effects of our deep transformative work. We are now actually looking at ourselves and the world around us from a new perspective.

This book demonstrates the inner workings of the grieving process. I provided the specific techniques for the practice of staying present and therefore available to transform your grief and encounter its strong emotions that fiercely challenge you. The tools are now at your fingertips; with focused awareness, you may methodically turn some of the seminal questions you've been asking yourself into concrete actions.

Through dealing with the suffering that is inherent during the grief journey, we have an opportunity to uncover our own true nature. Grief work is ultimately about challenging your assumptions about life: "Who am I without her? Where do I go after losing my home? Who am I now that I've been fired from my job? What does it mean that I'm still here now and he is gone?"

In the midst of sorrow, the blossoming of a new identity may mean many different things to you. Once you are no longer gripped by the old attachments, you become free to explore the deepest parts of yourself. As you ask yourself what you do and do not need, grief becomes the uncanny gateway to help gain the true knowledge of self.

Finding a New Identity After Loss

Identity consists mainly of our perceptions of ourselves based on the people and things we are attached to. When we lose them, we lose part of who we are. And yet life continues. Remember the feelings upon waking up in the immediate days and weeks following a profoundly huge loss? The body, moving in a robotic way, fighting against the lethargy of a tired mind, eyes barely open, two feet walking to the bathroom out of necessity?

Think of the body, the master survivor, maintaining life with the audacity to continue doing what it does. Despite our despair, despite our doubts, the amazing intelligence of our body is a powerful testament to the continuation of our existence.

Imagine a kitchen where you've cooked for the past twenty years, one with no ventilation, just tiny windows and a stove with slow, inefficient electric burners. One day the kitchen burns to the ground. Because you are hungry, because your body needs fuel, you need to continue cooking. Perhaps you can improvise and cook meals temporarily in the living room, or manage for a while on an outdoor grill, but the need for an indoor kitchen is painfully apparent, so you must rebuild it.

Is the new kitchen going to have ventilation or not? Big or small windows? Slow electric burners or quick and efficient gas burners? In order to define these details, you need to question your real needs and desires, likes and dislikes.

After all, you have cooked in that kitchen for years and are familiar with every detail, every nook and cranny. The memories of that kitchen may be overwhelmingly powerful to you, but now it is time to start imagining a new, more modern version that will serve your new needs.

Needs shift from basic survival instincts to those of a fuller, more spiritual vision of our life. Interestingly, many of us will gravitate to the familiar design of the old kitchen. But given time for reflection, new ideas and images will start to emerge that help us come closer to who we really are, and who we want to become.

Many of us identify who we are through our homes. Sometimes, the home is thought of as an extension of our physical bodies, something important to consider when working with grief. Identity is formed through what the body learns from its environment. The following two examples illustrate that.

Since a three-year-old cannot buy a car, rent a home, or find a job, the child must rely entirely on an adult caregiver. In this case, the father constantly puts down the three-year-old when he performs well. But complying with his father's expectations can be the difference between life and death. Consequently, the child learns either to become an underachiever or to hide his achievements so as not to upset his father.

The survival mechanism that informs the mind is deeply rooted in the wisdom of the body maintaining life at all costs. Putting our fingers in a live electric socket once gives the body enough information to avoid getting shocked again. The body has excellent cellular memory and keeps that survival mechanism alive. Even years later, while fixing a malfunctioning socket and knowing the power is off, your body still alerts you internally with caution signs warning of danger.

When defining ourselves after loss, it is very common to repeat old mechanisms, perform the same learned behaviors, and chant the same inner monologue because that is how we learned to survive. Repeating these behaviors grants us renewed suffering simply because our actions are antiquated and no longer match our present reality.

We must revisit the situation with new eyes, identifying our present needs and using our newly acquired skills—the ones lacking during the early formative years. Although old habits are difficult to change, respecting their power can actually be life affirming. We can see them in action and recognize them as a sign of the amazing intelligence of our bodies. Witnessing our broken heart's struggle to cope with the pain of loss and manage the accompanying symptoms of confusion and disorganized thinking is quite remarkable.

Isn't it a superbly opportune time to reimagine a new design when we no longer have the old kitchen, and yet our need for the food that's cooked in it is as real as the fire that consumed it? This is the opportunity hidden in the grief we experience. This is the transformative journey I'm talking about, the process that can take us from the void of devastation after loss to the fullness of a consciously lived life.

How Can the Transformation Be Accomplished?

My opinion is that the journey of discovery is threefold. Addressing the symptoms of our grief constitutes the first step. The second involves fully transiting the grieving process and achieving healthy resolution with it. The third entails reidentification based on our most intimate spiritual self. Having been stripped of our previous identity, laying bare the real core of who we are, we are now invited to approach the deepest parts of ourselves.

These three portions of the process of transformation are linked but not linear; simultaneously our awareness can shift as we sense some relief of our immediate symptoms. It is important to remember in grief work that any specific actions taken toward accomplishing resolution can be repeated and revisited at any point with renewed meaning.

The information you need comes as a result of your work and efforts to understand and relate to the experience at hand. This process involves observing your motivations, behaviors, and feelings. This book and the techniques proposed are designed to support you in the process of transforming your grief, offering practice as the foundation for the work. Using the tools you learned in chapter 4, you can reap the benefits you are after. Now, let's take a look at how each part of the process of transformation works.

The First Part: Addressing the Symptoms

How does addressing your symptoms help transform grief? Imagine yourself perched on a rolling hill, waiting to take in a beautiful sunset with some dear friends, when all of a sudden you are afflicted with a terrible toothache. Even if you are surrounded by love and support in the present moment, all you really want is to stop the pain; you need a dentist.

It is quite remarkable how, enticed by the presumption of the permanence of the body's vigor and endurance, we take our own health for granted.

A balanced body enhances your ability to transform grief. When the rug is pulled out from underneath you, shaking your foundation and threatening your stability, you can enter into a conversation with the body that will ultimately form the basis of your new identity. To regain presence for the process, you must address the different symptoms, particularly the physical ones.

The exercises contained in the program can help take care of the first part of the process by bringing the symptoms to a level of relative control. By practicing breath work, you become more present and aware and can help reestablish the normal rhythms of the body, finding ways of controlling your mental states and ultimately your new reality.

Practicing the Energy Flow Series assures the proper circulation of life force, avoiding blockages and facilitating free movement of consciousness within body and mind. The different *asanas* help get rid of the toxic chemical byproducts of pain and activate parts of the body where emotional issues tend to promote tension and stiffness. The specific actions performed in the Windmill bring your feelings to the surface of your awareness, allowing you to witness and identify them and ultimately to better understand how grief manifests in the body. Attitude of Discharging offers the increased charge of feelings and sensations of grief a way out. Concentrated Gazing promotes balance and better sleep.

The Self-Relaxation Technique helps combat the stressful effects of grief and diminishes general tension in the body, guiding you home to your normal sleep cycle. Resolve resets the mind so the body can manifest your deepest inner wishes, while Breath Meditation offers the calm stillness of body and mind that allows the Spirit to emerge more clearly.

All parts of the Yoga for Grief Relief *sadhana* prepare the body and the mind for the understanding of Spirit, which, as I've stated before, is the true source for the facilitation of grief.

The Second Part: Facilitating Grief

Facilitating grief implies making the experience of bereavement more manageable by following a road map such as the one proposed by J. William Worden in his Four Tasks of Mourning (2009). Employing the principles of yoga can assist in accomplishing those. Let's take a look at some additional guidelines.

Give yourself permission to grieve. Some people have a hard time accepting that grieving is appropriate. The reasons for these thoughts are often preconceived ideas about what to expose to others or how much time is acceptable to grieve. Personal difficulties such as the fear of being defined by grief, the possibility of feeling worse, or the chance you might trigger others' grief often prevent individuals from grieving.

If you care for grieving individuals and provide support, space, and resources, do you do the same for yourself? When flying on an airplane you are directed to put your oxygen mask on first in case of an emergency, before helping others. It is much the same in the grieving process—if you give yourself the permission to grieve first, you can then help others.

Provide yourself with the time you need to grieve. In the corporate world, employees are typically given a 72-hour "window" in which to grieve. Although there is no official time set to complete our grieving process, our minds tend to dictate that after one year has elapsed, "I should be done with my grief." Societal expectations, coupled with the pressure we put on ourselves to resume normal living, promote the belief that things will be much better in a year. Unfortunately, this unrealistic expectation is not only misleading, it is also counterproductive to maintaining a sense of hope.

For some of us, the second year of grief is even more difficult than the first. I encourage tolerance in allowing the time needed for working well with the complex grief experience. That permission alone is very important. In the normal course of bereavement, as time goes on, our grief frequently expresses itself as a

Sudden Temporary Upsurge of Grief (STUG; Rando 1993), sometimes related to and provoked by current life situations, other times showing up out of the blue. STUGs can provide us with a reflection of where we are in relation to our own grief. How fast we overcome it, how deep our feelings are felt, and how much our bodies are involved are all indicative of the skills we have developed, of the new pieces of information we have unveiled about ourselves.

It is necessary to mention that a prolonged time of coping with the disruptions of bereavement may be a marker for complicated grief, thus requiring specific interventions. All factors need to be taken into account to properly assess how and where we are in the very personal journey of grief.

Practice active listening with yourself. Have you ever had the experience of someone repeating back to you what they heard you say? Were you wide-eyed to hear the message repeated back? Did it sound like your thinking? Did you wonder, "Did I really say that?" This common occurrence happens in regular life as well as in therapeutic settings. A technique called "active listening," consisting of literally repeating a client's disclosure back to him or her, is frequently used to help clients reflect on the ways they name their own reality.

Consciously journaling our thoughts and experiences after yoga practice is a good way to allow the process of externalizing whatever comes to mind—unobstructed and uncensored. Look at your journal and repeat, "What I heard myself saying/thinking/feeling is..." Your reality is lived and determined by you in the way you talk about it and name it. How you do so determines how you live.

Resolve is a powerful tool for kick-starting the process of correcting unconscious habits and old behaviors. Another creative exercise uses free association to acquaint you with your true self by recording an audio version of feelings, emotions, and impressions. Listen to the recording and write, "What I heard myself saying is..." Just hearing your own voice, a more familiar expression of your inner dialogue offering insights, can evoke more powerful results.

Accept differences in the way you grieve. Trying to emulate a familial, societal, or cultural mold—in other words, forcing yourself into a preconceived form—may not serve you best. Grief is an intimate affair revealing the deeper self absolutely unique to each particular individual. Your way of grieving, the way you love, the things you love—they all speak to who you are. Find your way, honor it, and do it your way—even if it is very different from any expectations you might have or others may impose upon you.

Consider that your grief might change from one moment to another. You change just as the world around you changes, and, most important, the newly identified self feeds off of this. Welcome those changes; they reflect who you really are. You grieve each loss differently and you can even experience a multitude of polarized symptoms with one loss. Changes in the way you grieve express modifications in your mind and indicate that things are in fact reorganizing.

Even if things get more difficult, day in and day out, since everything changes, so too will that! Practice itself is an important monitor for assessing change. Identifying the different states of feeling and being aided by certain exercises or combinations thereof are part of the self-knowledge that grief unveils. What changed? What made the change? How can I reach that state again? These are some of the questions to ask yourself while viewing the many faces of your grieving process.

You must facilitate moving through your own grief—entirely, gently, and firmly—in your own unique way. Dr. Worden's four tasks are a pragmatic, user-friendly reference guide to evaluate the course of your grieving process and to locate yourself within that context. Next I offer you some suggestions of how to use yoga's knowledge and some of the techniques included in the *sadhana* to make your fulfillment of Worden's tasks appear less daunting.

ACCOMPLISHING ACCEPTANCE

Dr. Worden's four tasks, presented in chapter 1, are clear and direct. Find ways to accept the emotional reality of the loss (first task); process the pain of grief (second task); adapt to a new reality without the presence of the departed (third task); and relocate the lost person or object so you can embark on a new life (fourth task).

The yoga practice outlined in this book can be used to support your work on the tasks. For instance, remaining aware of the breath during Complete Breathing and witnessing without judgment any resistance you encounter can be instrumental in leading to accepting the reality of the loss.

Be aware of distracting behaviors, such as getting lost in a chain of thoughts, rushing to the computer, or grabbing the phone, which serve to avoid feeling the depth of what is happening. Tolerating the discomfort is a skillful way of meeting the unpleasant feelings of loss.

Journaling is one of the most widely used forms for reflective retelling of the facts. Going over the details again and recalling the events that happened is one of the most effective methods for gaining acceptance of loss. When journaling, the way you write about your reality is a reflection of the way you speak to yourself about it. When you relate the facts in your journal, also make sure you write about your feelings—it is of the essence. In order to do this you must identify and experience them, and to do so you must be present.

PROCESSING FEELINGS

In order to properly process feelings, we must first remain present for them. This is often one of the most difficult aspects of grieving, but it is also one of the most important. What does it mean to remain present? The actual practice of being present varies according to which feeling you focus on because feelings associated with grief vary widely and can be of different natures.

We often avoid our yoga practice, or falter when the techniques elicit a stronger perception of the feelings. Resistance is yet another sign of the struggle, so identify your options for staying present. Transiting your grief successfully and establishing ways to move out of the intense center of the experience to its quieter edges is the work. Since the only way out of the pain of grief is through it, you must enter and exit the process skillfully. Because of its passive nature, sadness—the most common feeling when grieving—allows us to actually sit with it. Most find sadness unpleasant and resist feeling it, so we put up defenses to elude it.

You can work on "sitting with sadness" simply by staying seated in meditation. While meditating, our minds tend to wander instead of focusing. That is true for our hearts as well; we tend to flee from sadness toward other feelings such as anger.

Anger is an active feeling and sitting with it can be extremely frustrating. It asks for mental and physical action. It is best processed when the target of the anger is identified and an effective method of expression is found. Anger is met with many societal judgments. We are taught that it is not a healthy feeling and that its expression makes others uncomfortable and only yields more anger. It is crucial to find an outlet for anger that does not conflict with what we have accepted as socially appropriate. Instead of aggression, I suggest considering assertiveness as an effective alternative way. You can forcefully push somebody away from your doorstep, or you can look straight into his eyes, pointing your finger at him while saying, "You do not walk into my house!" Through the practice of the Attitude of Discharging, anger can purposefully be expressed in the intimacy of your personal work. This technique offers modes of expression, from the more general involvement of the full body to the particular "aaah" sound that promotes vocalizing the active nature of the feeling. When not expressed outwardly, anger can turn inward resulting in self-destructive behaviors, such as relapsing with addictions. Sometimes anger can present itself as another feeling, such as guilt.

Because it is usually linked to irrational thoughts, guilt needs to be reality-tested in relation to the facts. Ask yourself if there is something you could have done differently, or if any actions taken could have indeed avoided the loss. Then you should be able to recognize whether you did or did not have any responsibility for how things happened. If you were indeed responsible, then what actions might help you to resolve the heavy burden of responsibility? If feelings of guilt still persist, what are they actually related to? What can the lesson learned be?

The palette of possible feelings is vast and unique to each individual. All feelings are valid—they are the elements the grieving heart is composed of and need to be processed so we can get to know ourselves better.

ADJUSTING TO THE NEW REALITY

Discovering how to adjust to a new reality varies distinctly according to the details of our life situation and how we interpret the meaning of the loss. The more the loss threatens our immediate survival, the more important it becomes to implement behaviors for adjustment.

For someone whose livelihood depended on who or what has been lost, finding ways to make ends meet and fulfill one's material obligations becomes of utmost importance. After our initial survival-based needs are met, other needs gain importance. These often manifest as questions that reflect the newly bereaved person's confusion or unfamiliarity with how to approach life after loss: "Who am I if not a married man? Who am I now that I am unemployed? Why continue to pray since my previous prayers were not answered?" By asking yourself these and other key questions, you learn who you have become and how to live more consciously without the deceased. As you embrace your new reality, the practice of Resolve is a solid ally imprinting new mental patterns and resetting old ones. Naming key resolutions such as "I pay my bills on time" or "I go to the gym every day" is what keeps the direction clear.

These mental adjustments become effective coping tools for the long-term experience of grief and bring immediate relief of present suffering. The dependence on the old reality starts to fade away. This offers a fresh, dynamic outlook that enhances independence and self-worth just by keeping a heightened and devoted focus on the newly blossoming self.

FACILITATING EMOTIONAL RELOCATION OF THE DECEASED OR LOST OBJECT

Yoga addresses the fundamental misapprehension of false ego identification: taking the impermanent for permanent. As you locate your place in the new reality, the relationship to who or what you have lost changes significantly. This clarification is essential for humbling the threatened ego. Instead of substituting the old attachment for a new one, seek a new place for yourself in relationship to who or what you lost. You can choose to focus on who you are now, without the departed person.

Breath Meditation is ideal for supporting the process of emotional relocation because it requires us tapping into our core issues, the profound aspects of our identity. For this deep and intimate work, our breath—our life force fueling our work—will continue to serve us until we too depart from this life.

Your previous identity, as effective and useful as it was, was linked to the past responses and behaviors relating to the world's challenges from a former, now-nonexistent time. The newly forming self-identity is being based on your revised inner world with more conscious thoughts, positive images, and appropriate needs that populate a healthier present. The focus of your embarkation is more savoring and embracing the actual internal journey leading you home to your true self, rather than the external aspects that previously defined your life.

DETACHED ATTACHMENT: A HEALTHY MODEL FOR THE FUTURE

After losing their son to an accident involving a drunk driver, the Smith family started a nonprofit organization to raise funds to create a public awareness campaign on the dangers of driving under the influence of alcohol.

The organization offered an outlet for their emotions and created a public forum for honoring the lost child in a meaningful way. The family seemed taken aback when I reminded them that the nonprofit too would one day come to an end. I explained that, for example, in the best-case scenario, their campaign would be 100 percent effective and no drunk drivers would exist, so no more funds would be needed.

My intention was to make the family aware of the finite nature of all things, including their organization. Even though they did not like anticipating the end, they were comforted when I asked them to consider this new piece of awareness as a gift from their son.

The ultimate intention of Worden's fourth task is to continue with the preexisting bond and to find ways of establishing an enduring connection with what we've lost. Interestingly enough, most existing models of grief therapy propose establishing new and healthier attachments as a way to continue with life.

I suggest you consider another way to look at this, one more closely related to the knowledge of yoga. I call it *detached attachment*, a very skillful tool. Do form attachments, yet keep full awareness of the fact that what you are attached to will inevitably disappear. Factoring in the truth of the impermanence of all things, you can establish new emotional bonds that empower you to live fully in the moment with no promise of tomorrow. Truly embodying this knowledge could effectively free you from remaining in the painful cycle of attachment. As all things eventually do, attachment too must end. Reassessing the value of holding on to a belief that only brings suffering leads us to ask, "Why not substitute it with a healthier, more reasonable concept that might feel even better?"

This approach bridges the pure and at times unattainable models of orthodox yoga with the accommodating processes of Western psychology. It offers a happy medium for making new attachments, which is an inherent need that humans have. By keeping a wide-open third eye, accessing a yogic awareness of the impermanence of all things, you still allow for loving fully. Loving in absence as well as in presence affords the opportunity of living fully with the guidance of the yogic principles for existence, reducing future suffering.

This is perhaps one of the most difficult challenges humans reckon with. We exhibit confusion, either mistaking love for attachment or struggling to love without it. The very core of the relocation process houses the seed of our new being. While relocating the deceased is the task, we too are finding a new emotional address for ourselves. Attributed to the universal integration of all existing things, balance equilibrates all systems simultaneously. Performing rituals and engaging in activities to honor the person or object we lost is, in truth, for us. The actual benefit gained is wholly for our healing; we can reclaim a sense of well-being while facilitating our adjustment process.

Revisiting the example of the Smith family, although the son might never see the nonprofit organization they opened in his name, the organization helped the family to find new purpose and a new identity.

The Third Part: Finding the New Identity

This is where the true gem lies, where the blessing in disguise is revealed. I am referring to the delight one feels when finding a pot of gold at the end of the rainbow. It is the result you are looking for when embarking on a conscious grief journey. You open a portal to a deeper connection with the Spirit, to the spiritual realm of your existence, by integrating fresh information on how the body processes grief with how the mind understands it.

When exploring this new connection, each person defines and relates to the Spirit in his or her own way. The quest to know the Spirit is age-old. Despite this book's many attempts to explain what Spirit is, and because Spirit is an experience, a practice might be worth a lot more than a thousand words. Let's use, yet again, another useful practice from yoga.

FINDING SPIRIT IN THE INNER SILENCE

I've found that practicing the first part of a technique called *antar mouna*, or "inner silence," is of much help when looking for a deeper connection with the Spirit. The technique consists of sitting in a comfortable position in stillness and with the eyes closed. Then hear all sounds, identifying loud ones from soft ones, distant ones from those that are close by, known ones from unknown ones.... Now switch your awareness to your ears—the outer ear, its temperature, its shape; try to feel the middle and even the inner ear. Perceive your ears....Now switch the awareness to You, the witness of the sounds—not the sounds, not the ears, but You, the witness of all sounds.

After mastering the technique using your ears, you may continue focusing on your feelings and then on your thoughts. This technique offers a gradual path toward the innermost self; it can be thought of as a system for disidentifying with the grosser planes of reality. The self we encounter is the one we are after.

The Spirit can be called the aspect of the being that witnesses life through a physical body; it is not the physical body, nor the facts of the experience. It is the observer that is not altered by what it observes, just as a mirror is not affected by the items it reflects.

SKILLFUL QUESTIONING

Finding the new identity can be greatly helped by using one of the golden tools in yoga: *atma vichara*, or self-inquiry. The essential question of the inquiry is, "Who am I?" The answer can only be found within, by connecting with the witness, by asking the observer within, by getting to know your own Spirit.

The question is intended to help you connect with the "subject" of this existence, or the "I." We identify ourselves by the states we go through, the things we possess, and the objects we relate to. Answers such as "I am rich" or "I am sad" lead to a false identification.

The kind of self-inquiry I'm indicating is best conducted when working on discarding the object-based identity—what I am—in order to discover the subject-based one: who I am. It is a quest for the true self in all that we do, in every thought, every speech, every action.

The reason to perform self-inquiry is that we don't purport to know who we are, and grief offers us plenty to doubt. The skillful questioning is not just related to what family you belong to or which country you were born in; rather it seeks to unmask your essential identity as an embodied Spirit. That part of yourself, as it relates to "I," is not identified with the physical.

It connects you with the pure awareness of who you are rather than what you are aware of. Bear in mind that the difference between object and subject appears subtle to us and that we are inherently confused about these two realms. Other clarifying questions are: Who is feeling sad? Who is experiencing anxiety? Who is feeling lonely and fearful? Most grievers do not want to be defined by their grief: this technique helps connect with the one witnessing the suffering, not the suffering itself.

COGNITIVE REFRAMING

Vicki Panagotacos (2012, 292), a gifted American grief therapist, proposes four essential questions to guide the process of envisioning a new self and a new life by defining certain parameters most of us need to deal with. I've found that her questions are skillful in supporting a griever's practice of *atma vichara*, or self-inquiry. The four questions are as follows:

1. What do you want to include in your life?

2. What don't you want to include in your life?

3. What do you have in your life that you want to eliminate?

4. What do you have in your life that you want to keep?

Panagotacos proposes writing down the answers, one each on separate pages. In her therapy practice she dedicates a session to providing a final list to her clients, including the answers to question 1, plus the "converted answers" to questions 2, 3, and 4. (For example, "I don't want to move" converts to "I want to stay where I am living" [293]). I suggest you convert your answers to questions 2, 3, and 4, then write a document with your final list. These are great questions to ask yourself to promote awareness of your personal journey and to find yourself in your new life plans.

According to Karen Whitley Bell, who wrote *Living at the End of Life: A Hospice Nurse Addresses the Most Common Questions* (2010), one of the most common comments of dying individuals when asked about what they regret about their lives is that they wish they would have lived more according to their desires than others' expectations. While our lives can only be breathed through our own nostrils, sometimes we adopt other people's beliefs about what's best for us and assume them as guiding lights. It is only through fulfilling the needs and the deep desires of our hearts that we can achieve our destiny, flowing in the universal order of all existing things.

A tree does not develop branches just for birds to perch; rather, because the branches form that is in the nature of the tree's development and unfolding. The fact that a bird can perch on its branch is just so, and not the tree's reason for being.

If your previous identity was based on others' needs, you can now redesign and redefine anew by accessing one of humanity's essential desires: "the desire for purpose, the drive to become who you are meant to be," as expressed by Rod Stryker (2011, 35). "Your long-term happiness and fulfillment," he continues, "depend on your ability to fulfill your personal *dharma* and fill the place in the world that only you can fill."

What Are the Possible Meanings of Finding a New Identity After Loss?

One of the amazing features of the human brain is its ability to assign meaning to our experiences. This is due to the presence of the neocortex: a vast net of interconnected neurons that complement the functions of the reptilian brain, interacting with the limbic system and the emotional brain. This emotional part of the brain appeared in mammals only just a few million years ago. So what does this process of transformation mean for an individual? There is no shortage of meanings!

Finding a Light at the End of the Tunnel

Despair is common in grief because sometimes, in the vast darkness of the process, we cannot envision how life could possibly go on. It is like being stuck in a dark tunnel, unable to sense light at the other end.

This metaphor often refers to the impossibility of identifying a solution or resolution for an existing situation when we are in the thick of it. Existence continues after loss, and so can we. By trusting that there is light somewhere and that the darkness in which we are immersed in the present moment will not be there forever, we can relax knowing that, in time, it too will change like everything else does.

The case of one of my clients, Joan, comes to mind. Feeling bored practicing Concentrated Gazing, she asked me to use a lit candle for the distant focal point instead of a black dot. Her assumption was that the dancing flame would prevent her from feeling drowsy.

Because she had defined the experience of her grief as walking through a dark tunnel with no end, I proposed to keep this image in mind as she practiced. This conscious "shifting" of attention from her present reality of pain and confusion to the promise of an enlightened future served as a powerful metaphor for Joan. Performing this form of Concentrated Gazing, she took this metaphor of the light at the end of the tunnel to the physical realm of her practice.

Focusing the eye on the distant object became a symbol of her willingness to face the unknown future, projecting her intention to move beyond the present feelings of pain, confusion, and isolation. Even though we might be mired in darkness and despair, the arc of our vision carries us to a deeper reality, one from which we emerge stronger and wiser. Thanks to this conscious work we are able to overcome the negative anticipatory thinking that has ensnared us.

While teaching a class at the University of California–Berkeley, I once heard a seasoned therapist share her newly found observation. She stated that after thirty-five years of counseling clients, she saw that all therapeutic work is based in dealing with grief!

Although most grieving individuals certainly would prefer a quick fix, those who chose to laboriously engage in grief work can find hope, regain trust, and reduce their pain. Enticed by the possibility of a better life, one more abundant in light and self-love, they realize that just on the other side of the veil of darkness is so much more than most of us ever thought possible. We envision the positive outcome of our grief work: a torch that blazes at the other side with the newly discovered knowledge of self.

Experiencing Rebirth

Sometimes the experience of arriving to a new self is so intense that people refer to it as a new birth or a rebirth. This is something I've seen happen particularly in the case of cancer patients. People facing cancer have a primary loss of health, but they also face secondary losses such as the loss of the ability to perform familiar activities, or the loss of hair due to chemotherapy's secondary effects.

Once losses have been normalized, a surprising number of cancer patients express enjoying newly cherished aspects of life. They have reported feeling deeper gratitude, delighting in delicate interpersonal contact, embodying a deeper knowing of their personal needs, and more actively participating in increased compassionate self-care.

Many perceive this as a new life. Often cancer patients will refer to the date of diagnosis as a kind of "second birthday."

THE MYTH OF THE PHOENIX

The phoenix: a mythical bird that obtains new life by rising from the ashes of its predecessor. The aftermath of the shocking devastation of loss is described using imagery referring to scorched landscapes after a fire: empty, colorless, vacant, dark, and lifeless. Using this metaphor, imagine what this charred landscape, home to so many different animals, plants, and trees might have contained before. The ashes contain the recorded imprint of the preexisting fauna and flora as well as the elements that help the soil become more fertile and that improve the overall health of the forest. Despite the absence of what was lost, their memory is retained concentrated in the ash, which fertilizes the forest floor and facilitates regrowth.

By remaining present for the feelings that come up in grief, we become like the phoenix, created anew from the ashes left behind by loss. In her beautiful short piece on the loss of a son-in-law, Kimberley Pittman-Schulz writes that "to grieve one death means always to grieve two" (2011, 16). This is true for so many of the people hollowed out by their experience of loss. Whatever time it takes—months or years—to become aware of how deeply a loss has penetrated us, we have the option of living in honor of the departed or deceased by following our path.

The myth of the phoenix is a powerful one for understanding how, from the depths of the ashes, a new being is born, rising high above the place of our sorrow and despair, endowed with new perspectives and acquired wisdom.

Honoring the Legacy of the Departed

Other than profoundly negative relationships, the severance of which provides relief, most of us want to continue the bonds, finding ways to honor the legacy of what we have lost.

Mostly, we choose to believe that the departed would prefer us to be happy and to still fulfill our dreams. In doing so, this becomes a way of honoring the memory and intentions of the departed, and a way of staying in contact with them. It provides us with a fresh opportunity to share our new information about ourselves and our accomplishments with the deceased in a figurative way that we believe would make them happy.

It allows our bodies to engage in an action, the simple action of living our lives in a better way. We cannot touch the hand of a lost child or physically hug a lost pet, yet we find new endeavors to accomplish "in honor of," "as related to," and "in the name of" the departed, bringing new meaning to the loss.

This can serve us by acknowledging and attending to the unfinished business, and still effect perceptive changes, even in our relationship with the deceased.

Being an Example to Others

Our society is not comfortable with grief, nor does it offer suitable outlets for expression of the related feelings. Instead, grief often gets swept under the rug. A common belief is that we get over our grief with the passage of time. Nothing could be further from the truth: there is no "getting over" our grief, and it does not simply fade away with time. By being patient with our own process, we teach others patience. By consciously addressing our symptoms, we teach others about self-care. By properly naming our feelings and speaking our truth, we teach others to hear grievers out and console them.

Finding a new identity after loss requires awareness and presence for the multitude of insights grief offers. By doing our work and sharing our experience we become a model, an example that others can benefit from in their own lives. Society loves those characters who are secure, solid, assertive, and exhibit dominion over uncertainties. Everyone gravitates toward the hero who humbly understands personal weaknesses, has self-reliant qualities, and has integrated acquired knowledge and wisdom.

As we transit the grieving process from our hearts and the intricacies of our minds, we discover our resilience and strengthen our skills, defining a better life and setting a good example to be witnessed by others.

Learning New Ways of Loving

Our new identity can offer a different relationship between love and attachment, one that moves away from presenting them as equal. I once heard a noted professional say that grief is the price we pay for love, but in truth grief is the price we pay for attachment.

To differentiate love from attachment we set a new standard of possibility, both with others and for ourselves. Societies flourishing in balance and truth start with individuals, and right now that is you and me.

By making love and attachment the same, we mistake the impermanent for permanent; and instead of loving unconditionally, we create the conditions for codependence. By understanding how to continue loving in the face of absence, we liberate love from its material basis, and liberate ourselves in the process. Then love achieves its full force, becoming capable of transforming in unexpected ways, undoing the old, and granting us access to a new way of loving ourselves with freedom and respect.

Sinking into the Order of the Universe

The universal order is already in existence, and sinking into it promotes actions that reinforce the principle of pronoia, which dictates that the universe is conspiring in your highest good in both the internal and external worlds. The acceptance of this fact reestablishes our trust in life and brings a sense of hope that is elusive while in grief.

Change is a constant force in the order of the universe. As you become aware of personal choices that no longer serve you, trusting the universal force activates conscious envisioning of new, more appropriate options. Another essential yogic truth expresses that "all the knowledge you need for your life is already within you." Considering this can help you break free from previously held beliefs that cause resistance.

In doing so, you remove the first of the five causes of suffering as stated by Patanjali in *The Yoga Sutras*: ignorance of the truth. Replacing ignorance with knowledge based on our present reality is of tangible benefit to grievers.

The resulting feeling is similar to what we experience when we swim with the current or when we sleep at night: a sense of going with the flow characterized by comfort and ease. That does not mean the absolute absence of struggle. It suggests that as we practice, we encounter accommodating moments that allow us to get comfortable along with the discomfort, or relax within the unrest, feeling ease in the midst of complexity.

You recognize that you are part of a larger organism abundant in activity and pulsating with life. The acceptance that you are part of a community of others who have hopes, desires, and fears just like you do can be a powerful antidote to the paralyzing isolation of grief.

You can change an identity established on the old model of attachments and embrace a new one based on the synchronicity of your coexistence with the universe. Most of the work in yoga is related to understanding this union and allowing it to be life's guiding light. Transforming our grief offers the opportunity most of us seek to access: to bathe in the universal wisdom and become part of the whole. This experience changes our life forever, in the intimacy of our solitude or in the company of the rest of humanity.

Grief is without a doubt the most intense invitation to acknowledge the union of all existing things I have known. It not only forces us to live with amazingly contradictory feelings and emotions, such as "I don't want to ever think of him again—I don't want to ever forget him," but also because we are prompted to go through extremely opposite conditions in our bodies as well: from feeling full of energy when experiencing the initial shock of a loss to feeling deep fatigue a few days later. As confusing as these extremes might seem to our minds, our hearts find solace and relief when able to link these opposing feelings and thoughts with the word "and." A significant part of the new identity results from substituting the limiting "but" for a more inclusive "and." Just think of how different it feels to hear yourself saying, "I want to remarry but no other woman will love me the same way" versus "I want to remarry and no other woman will love me the same way." The very presence of the word "but" is divisive, separating, not conducive to reconciliation—qualities that grievers need no more of. On the contrary, "and" is inclusive, uniting, an invitation to reconcile. These are all milestones for a griever along his or her journey through grief.

As we conclude the discussion of how to transform grief into a source of self-knowledge toward a new identity, I would like to revive the image of a windmill as a metaphor for this process of transformation. Just as the windmill blades are moved by wind, our whole being is swept up by the mystery of loss. This natural phenomenon is what sparks the transformation of hard grains into edible flour, just as loss forces us to transform the depths of who we are. The newly created flour is the starting point of a future meal, just as the newly acquired knowledge we have gained from loss is the starting point of a new "I."

Conclusion

"Solitude has soft, silky hands, but with strong fingers it
grasps the heart and makes it ache with sorrow. Solitude is the
ally of sorrow as well as a companion of spiritual exaltation."

—Kahlil Gibran (2005, 59)

Grief affects us on the deepest level imaginable in all aspects of our humanity: the physical, mental, and spiritual. Because so much of our identity is wrapped up in previous attachments, whether good or bad, that identity is stripped away when we lose those persons or objects to which we've become attached. They often loom so largely in our world that we rarely take time to question how our lives might be affected by their absence. When that moment comes, we are forced to answer that question. Regardless of our cultural background or religious affiliation we feel that unique sensation that comes with loss. Beyond any name we can find for it, our whole being "knows" what we are going through.

This book is born from that feeling deep within me; it is one more expression of how my grief permeated my actions, thoughts, and words. I now realize that fully embracing my personal grief, along with my passion for working with griev-ers professionally, has been a way of emotionally relocating my mother, and, inev-itably, myself. The "I" speaking to you in the pages of this book could not exist without first having transformed my own grief.

I've shared information about many aspects of grief that can help you normal-ize yours. Please know that loss is part of the human condition and, sooner or later, grief is felt by all. Understanding how East and West differ in their view of grief may help you tolerate your contradicting feelings and thoughts. Your present reality is, in a way, induced by your brain. Be patient: all throughout life, your brain adapts by rewiring itself through experience—so can you!

I've offered tools to transform your physical reality through body movements and postures, as well as to reshape your mental panorama through breath work and connect with the deep wisdom of your Spirit through meditation. I've given suggestions to tailor your practice according to your abilities and needs. Understanding the relationship between the techniques and the ways the tech-niques affect grief can inform your choices as to which of them to practice.

The simple act of practicing is more important than any one specific exercise contained in this book. What helps you most is proving to yourself that you have the intention to change. Practice will help you find ways of keeping an enduring connection with who or what has departed while relating to your new emerging self. As you witness yourself, the practice has already begun.

Through the power of yoga, you are able to plunge into the depths that house not only your pain but also your true self. It is often during this time that we are able to make real, lasting changes that put us on a new path toward greater self-fulfillment and ultimate acceptance of the laws of the Universe—our humble essence is just one more grain of sand on the shores of existence.

In our modern society, we tend to trek through life at a breakneck pace, stop-ping to look and listen only rarely, either when it's convenient or, most common, when we are shocked into awareness. Loss itself causes the soul-stirring awaken-ing that transforms us, even though grief asks not if we are prepared for such transformative work.

Time is an essential part of the process, just not the only one. Paying close attention to the wisdom of our Spirit is required. Bereavement is a time when the

Spirit can be contacted most readily because its latent power is clearly accessible. As you transcend the apparent duality of existence you will find that life and death, absence and presence, are part of one continuum and cannot strip you of the love residing underneath your suffering.

The yoga practice I've shared with you is not to help avoid suffering; rather, it is to aid you in finding relief. As you experience your grief more fully, you move closer to the unique being that you truly are. Grief then becomes a naturally humbling invitation to self-reflection, not something to be reviled or shunned. Many cultures accept death as a time of renewal, as a precious moment that teaches us about the bonds we all share, including the one with oneself. When loss occurs, many of us let in loneliness for the first time. As you acknowledge the life that has departed you also feel the life that still resides within, and you are invited to recognize that, one day, this life will too depart.

This is your time to access a sacred space, set your intentions, and witness the unfolding of life: one breath in, one breath out. You are the one who needs acknowledgment in this moment more than anything else. Here, yoga can once again assist you! Just consider one of yoga's core teachings: "What we are looking for is the one who is looking." You are on your way...

Glossary

Asana

Physical movement or posture traditionally found in the system of yoga. By first addressing the physical, *asanas* help establish a strong foundation in the body before more advanced exercises and meditation are performed.

Attachment theory

Theory pioneered by the behaviorist John Bowlby that discusses how we as human beings form emotional bonds as infants and children that then determine our love-related behaviors into adulthood.

Ayurveda

A science of life, *ayur* meaning life and *veda* meaning science or knowledge. It offers a body of wisdom designed to help people stay vital while realizing their full human potential. Providing guidelines on ideal daily and seasonal routines, Ayurveda reminds us that health is the balanced and dynamic integration of our environment, mind, body, and spirit.

Chakras

Energetic centers in the physical body that correspond to different nerve plexuses and endocrine glands as well as certain emotional and psychological traits. Each chakra signifies different stages of human evolution.

Degriefing process

An integrated approach to grief therapy pioneered by Lyn Prashant that incorporates bodywork, traditional grief counseling, and complementary therapies.

J. William Worden

American psychologist and grief counselor who created the "tasks" model of grieving, which identifies four tasks the griever must transit to fulfill a normal grieving process.

Meditation

Meditation is identified by Patanjali, who wrote *The Yoga Sutras of Patanjali*, as the primary means by which the practitioner achieves liberation. It usually entails limiting the range of change of the mind to bring about calm and focus.

Normalization

The concept encountered in grief therapy that grief symptoms are normal, and that the suffering a griever feels after a loss is not to be shunned. It takes into account both cultural and familial dismissals of grief. This is often a way for grievers to first accept the reality of their loss and to start processing through the pain of their grief.

Pranayama

Breathing exercises traditionally found in the system of yoga. By manipulating the *prana* (life force), *pranayama* leads us to operate on the consciousness itself.

Primary loss

The loss of a loved one, object, or ideal that occurs first and causes a typical grief reaction.

Psychophysiology

Multidisciplinary study of psychology, biology, and neurology that demonstrates how environmental factors influence us on a psychological level.

Sadhana

A spiritual practice that advocates a set of practical exercises to establish regularity that, sustained over time, leads us to spiritual fulfillment.

Sankalpa

The yogic principle of Resolve. This helps aid practitioners in identifying and setting goals for their practice and, therefore, their lives.

Secondary losses

Losses that occur as a result of the primary loss having occurred.

Shatkarma

Cleansing exercises that help purify both the body and mind, preparing the practitioner for meditation.

Yoga

A six-thousand-year-old discipline from ancient India, whereby through physical exercises, breath work, and meditation, we can overcome the suffering we encounter in life and contact our Spirit.

Yoga chikitsa

Man's first attempt at unitive understanding of the mind, emotions, and physical distress, and the oldest holistic concept and therapy in the world.

Yoga therapy

Western modulation of the original discipline of yoga, often performed one-on-one, that combines traditional therapeutic models with the benefits bestowed by the practice of yoga.

References

Begley, Sharon. 2007. "The Brain: How the Brain Rewires Itself." *Time*, January 19, 2007. http://content.time.com/time/magazine/article/0,9171,1580438,00.html.

Bhaktivedanta, A. C. Swami Prabhupada. 1972. *Bhagavad-Gita as It Is.* Los Angeles: Bhaktivedanta Book Trust.

Boleyn-Fitzgerald, Miriam. 2010. *Pictures of the Mind: What the New Neuroscience Tells Us About Who We Are.* New York: FT Press.

Bowlby, John. 1969. *Attachment and Loss: Vol. 1. Attachment.* New York: BasicBooks.

Bowlby, John. 1972. *Attachment and Loss: Vol. 2. Separation: Anxiety and Anger.* New York: BasicBooks.

Brezsny, Rob. 2009. *Pronoia Is the Antidote for Paranoia, Revised and Expanded: How the Whole World is Conspiring to Shower You with Blessings.* Berkeley, CA: North Atlantic Books.

Broberg, Anders G. 2000. "A Review of Interventions in the Parent–Child Relationship Informed by Attachment Theory." *Acta Pædiatrica* 89 (434): 37–42.

Bryant, Edwin F., ed. 2009. *The Yoga Sutras of Patanjali: A New Edition, Translation, and Commentary.* New York: Farrar, Straus and Giroux.

Davidson, Richard. 2012. *The Emotional Life of Your Brain: How Its Unique Patterns Affect the Way You Think, Feel, and Live—and How You Can Change Them.* New York: Hudson Street Press.

Diamond, Lisa M. 2001. "Contributions of Psychophysiology to Research on Adult Attachment: Review and Recommendations." *Personality and Social Psychology Review* 5 (4): 276–95.

Diemer, Deedre. 1998. *The ABCs of Chakra Therapy: A Workbook.* York Beach, Maine: Samuel Weiser, Inc.

Freud, Sigmund. 1953. "Mourning and Melancholia." In *Collected Papers, Vol. IV,* edited by Ernest Jones. 152–70. London: The Hogarth Press.

Gardner, James. 2002. "Somatic Aspects of Loss and Grief." Notes for U.C. Berkeley Extension Continuing Education Workshop, Berkeley, Calif., October 26–27.

Gardner, James. 2010. "The Anxiety Toolbox Program." http://www.anxietytool box.com/toolbox/index.htm.

Gibran, Kahlil. 2005. "Silent Sorrow." In *The Kahlil Gibran Reader: Inspirational Writings,* translated by Anthonly R. Ferris. 59–61. New York: Citadel Press.

Goethe, Johann Wolfgang von (attributed). Date unknown. From "Until One Is Committed..." by Meredith Lee, Goethe Society of North America, last modified March 5, 1998. http://www.goethesociety.org/pages/quotescom. html.

Lowen, Alexander. 1994. *Bioenergetics: The Revolutionary Therapy That Uses the Language of the Body to Heal the Problems of the Mind.* New York: Penguin/Arkana.

Lunche, Howard J. 1999. *Understanding Grief: A Guide for the Bereaved.* Berkeley, CA: SVL Press.

Main, Mary, and Judith Solomon. 1986. "Discovery of an Insecure Disoriented Attachment Pattern: Procedures, Findings and Implications for the Classification of Behavior." In *Affective Development in Infancy*, edited by T. Berry Brazelton and Michael Yogman. New York: Ablex Publishing.

Panagotacos, Vicki. 2012. "Defining and Envisioning Self." In *Techniques of Grief Therapy: Creative Practices for Counseling the Bereaved*, edited by Robert A. Neimeyer. New York: Routledge.

Pascual-Leone, Alvaro. 2001. "The Brain That Plays Music and Is Changed By It." *Annals of the New York Academy of Sciences* 930: 315–29.

Pert, Candace. 1997. *Molecules of Emotion: Why You Feel the Way You Feel*. New York: Scribner.

Pittman-Schulz, Kimberley. 2011. "Light, Held Together By Water." *The Sun Magazine*, October 16, 2011.

Prashant, Lyn. 2002. *The Art of Transforming Grief: A Practical Guide for Combining Conventional and Complementary Mind-Body Therapies*. San Anselmo, Calif.: Self-published.

Prashant, Lyn. 2005. Keynote speech at the 12th Annual National Alzheimer's Conference, Mayo Clinic, Rochester, Minn., November.

Rando, Therese. 1993. *Treatment of Complicated Mourning*. Champaign, Ill.: Research Press.

Rawat, Prem Pal Singh. 1990, March 16. Lecture at The Prem Rawat Foundation, Buenos Aires, Argentina.

Reich, Wilhelm. 1949. *Character Analysis*. New York: Farrar, Straus, and Giroux.

Rosenbaum Bent, and Sverre Varvin. 2007. "The Influence of Extreme Traumatization on Body, Mind and Social Relations." *International Journal of Psychoanalysis* 88(6): 1527–42.

Satyananda, Swami. 1976. *Four Chapters on Freedom*. Bihar, India: Yoga Publications Trust.

Satyananda, Swami. 1985. *Kundalini Tantra*. Bihar, India: Yoga Publications Trust.

Selby, John. 1992. *Kundalini Awakening: A Gentle Guide to Chakra Activation and Spiritual Growth*. New York: Bantam Books.

Stryker, Rod. 2011. *The Four Desires: Creating a Life of Purpose, Happiness, Prosperity, and Freedom*. New York: Delcorte Press.

Subramuniyaswami, Sivaya. 1999. *Weaver's Wisdom: Ancient Precepts for a Perfect Life*. Kapaa, HI: Himalayan Academy.

Ulvestad, Elling. 2012. "Psychoneuroimmunology: The Experiential Dimension." *Methods in Molecular Biology* 934: 21–37.

Van den Berg, Bellis., Albert Wong, Peter van der Velden, Hendriek Boshuizen, and Linda Grievink. 2012. "Disaster Exposure as a Risk Factor for Mental Health Problems, Eighteen Months, Four and Ten Years Post-Disaster: A Longitudinal Study." *BMC Psychiatry* 12: 147–60.

Whitley Bell, Karen. 2010. *Living at the End of Life: A Hospice Nurse Addresses the Most Common Questions*. New York: Sterling Publishing.

Weintraub, Amy. 2004. *Yoga for Depression: A Compassionate Guide to Relieve Suffering Through Yoga*. New York: Broadway Books.

Worden, J. William. 2009. *Grief Counseling and Grief Therapy: A Handbook for the Mental Health Practitioner*. 4th ed. New York: Springer Publishing Co.

Antonio Sausys, MA, IGT, CMT, RYT, is a somatic psychotherapist and yoga instructor specializing in one-on-one yoga therapy for people with chronic and acute medical conditions, as well as emotional imbalance. He studied with yoga masters and teachers such as Indra Devi, Swami Maitreyananda, and Larry Payne. He has continued his professional development with training in integrative grief therapy with Lyn Prashant, foot reflexology, Swedish therapeutic massage, and Reiki. Antonio teaches and lectures periodically at the University of California, Berkeley; at the California Institute of Integral Studies, Kripalu Center for Yoga and Health. He is a member of the World Yoga Council, the International Association of Yoga Therapists, and the Association for Death Education and Counseling. He is the founder and executive director of Yoga for Health—the International Yoga Therapy Conference, and television host for *YogiViews*. For more information, visit yogaforgriefrelief.com.

The author thanks his freelance editor, **Elliott Vogel**, for his creative assistance on *Yoga for Grief Relief*. Vogel is a freelance writer and editor. A student of yoga for over ten years, Vogel's journey studying the philosophy and practice of yoga originated under the tutelage of the book's author, Antonio Sausys. He currently resides in Mill Valley, CA.

Foreword writer **Lyn Prashant, PhD, FT, IGT, SYVC**, is a somatic thanatologist, certified grief counselor, massage therapist, yoga instructor, author, and international presenter. She is the director and founder of Degriefing® (Integrative Grief Therapy) and the Institute of Somatic Thanatology.

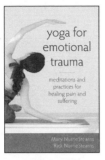
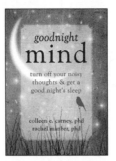
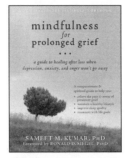
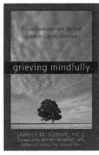
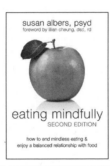
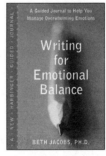
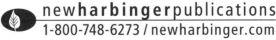